*William J. Fay*

# AIDS
# The Spiritual Dilemma

## *John E. Fortunato*

**Harper & Row, Publishers, San Francisco**

Cambridge, Hagerstown, New York, Philadelphia, Washington
London, Mexico City, São Paulo, Singapore, Sydney

For Jack Balcer,

who has shown me that a full life
has nothing to do with its length.

**Library of Congress Cataloging-in-Publication Data**

Fortunato, John E.
   AIDS, the spiritual dilemma.

   1. AIDS (Disease)—Religious aspects—Christianity.
I. Title.
RC607.A26F67   1987        248.8'6        86–43006
ISBN 0-06-250338-3 (pbk.)

90  91        10  9  8  7  6

# Contents

In writing stories of persons in counseling, psychotherapy, or spiritual direction, I have not used specific individuals but have created composites for illustrative purposes.

# Preface

It doesn't matter from what angle you look: AIDS is a terrible thing. And it is going to be with us for a long time.

Even if a vaccine were developed tomorrow, the number of people already infected is enormous. Even if a cure were found today, the number of dead is great, and the effect on all those whose lives indirectly have been touched by this dreadful illness will last for decades. How can we bear the pain of this development in world history? How can we deal with AIDS and not either engage in full-scale denial or be immobilized? It is my conviction that the only way out is to go deeper.

This is a book about the meaning of AIDS. It is an attempt to plumb the depths of AIDS and the impact it has had, is having, and will continue to have on our lives. As the words *The Spiritual Dilemma* suggest, I have attempted in these pages to look *beneath* the medical, psychological, sociological, and even pastoral facts, and to try to glimpse the reality of AIDS in its broadest context.

As a believing person, I see this "broadest context" as the spiritual realm—the dimension of being from which all meaning emanates, the cosmic context in which all reality is grounded. To the extent that we are willing to explore these mostly hidden recesses of our souls, I am convinced we shall achieve peace with this disease. It is my hope that what follows will help us on that part of our journey.

This book is not only for people who have the disease; AIDS affects each of us. No exceptions. The universe in which we live is different now. It has been irrevocably changed. One's being in a low-risk group is of no consequence in this regard. The meanings of things all around us have been transformed by AIDS. To ignore these alterations would be to play the ostrich. And in all candor, we cannot afford to do that.

AIDS, contrary to popular opinion, is not a gay disease. It is not a disease that only gay people can contract (as is the case with black people and sickle cell anemia). Nor is it a disease that was started by gay people; there is no evidence that gay people *brought* AIDS to the United States. Nor is it a disease that was caused by gay people; we did not, by virtue of being homosexual, somehow spawn this virus.

It is true that most of the initial cases of AIDS reported in the United States appeared in the gay community (more than 80 percent). The reasons for that demographic skew are various. But the monopoly has long since been undone. And what is more, in other countries, notably Africa, AIDS is and has all along been predominantly a heterosexual disease primarily affecting women and children . . . which has its own psycho-social impact.

Nevertheless, I am going to be writing about AIDS mostly from a gay perspective. Why?

I have followed a piece of advice a former mentor

repeatedly gave me as I wrote my first book, *Embracing the Exile: Healing Journeys of Gay Christians*. "Write about the *spiritual journey*," he would say, "and use the gay stuff—which is closest to home for you—for your most poignant illustrations."

It was good advice. More than half of the 500 or so letters I have received since *Embracing*'s publication have been from nongay people who were moved not by associations with gay friends or relatives, but by associations with *their own experience of exile* (as, for instance, divorced, unmarried, handicapped, or ethnic people).

AIDS is a disease anyone can get. But my fifteen friends who have died of it, and the psychotherapy patients or spiritual directees whom I have seen through it to the end, and those I currently see, are almost all gay. I again have tried to write about the spiritual journey, in particular as it relates to AIDS. I know it mostly from a gay point of view. If that is not *your* context, you may be inclined to generalize from *mine*. All the better.

My second reason for dealing with AIDS mostly in a gay context is that society has so tightly associated AIDS with gay men. As noted above, this identification is unfounded. That in itself is of enormous spiritual consequence and has profound spiritual meaning. To ignore this association would be to miss a major signpost pointing toward the profoundest reaches of AIDS's meaning.

A word about God-language. Harper & Row graciously has allowed me in this book to observe two unusual linguistic conventions. First, I have followed the older usage of initial capital letters in pronouns referring to God, as in *He*, *Him*, and *His*. The more modern convention of using lowercase initial letters for these pronouns is mostly a secular, scholarly development. The capitals were perceived by academics as subjective and reverential; the university strives to be objective. The use of an initial cap H was construed as making a "faith statement" that was felt to be inappropriate in the purportedly "neutral" environment of academia. The convention now has been applied to almost all religious books.

I prefer not to follow this newer convention for several reasons. First, this is not an academic book; it is quite devotional. But even if this *were* a purely scholarly work, I find that I at least try to be reverent *all* the time, even when I write books. I cannot imagine what it might mean to stand outside my faith and frankly, I am suspect of those academicians who claim, in their research, to leave their beliefs aside. (I prefer those who state their biases straightforwardly at the outset and then proceed.)

Moreover, I perceive the use of lowercase initial letters for pronouns referring to God as anything but neutral; it is very much a "faith statement." In this modern theological era, pervaded by the illusion of scientific objectivity, using He and Him—especially in relation to Jesus in His earthly life—has become embarrassing. Earthly divinity is a notion "enlightened" Christians prefer to downplay in their prose, and using the lowercase H lets one off the hook. This is no neutral stance.

But I stand firmly in the Catholic faith embodied in

the Anglican tradition. I make no apology for believing that Jesus of Nazareth was true God and true man. How, then, could I not want to show Him reverence?

The second deviation from usual convention that Harper & Row has permitted me to make is that, except when referring to Jesus, I have alternately used masculine and feminine pronouns—both He and She, Him and Her—when speaking of God. While this may seem daring to some, I have done it simply to be accurate. If God is not the totality both of masculinity and feminity—*anima* and *animus*—we are all in trouble. I cannot any longer, in good conscience, ignore half of this reality in my prose. So if the use of both genders is distracting to you at first, I ask your forbearance: God our Mother has been waiting in the wings a long time.

I am grateful to many people who have seen me through the birthing of this book. To John, my life-mate, whose historical knowledge and logical prowess helped keep my intuitive, impulsive literary inclinations within reasonable bounds, I am deeply indebted. I suspect you should be, too. I would also like to thank Janice Johnson, my editor at Harper & Row, with whom editing has been a wonderful, deepening dialogue. And warm thanks go also to my curate and friend, Mother Joy Rogers. Joy's heart dwells so much in the same corner of the universe as mine that she was able to be the most crystal clear mirror I could have hoped for as I refined my thoughts and words.

For my many spiritual friends who have encouraged me on my path, I thank God. If this book says anything of importance, it will be because my consciousness was formed by loving, insightful soul mates who enabled me to *be* in places I would otherwise have left unexplored. And for my patients, who show me the healing power of God, each week filling me with awe and hope, I also give thanks.

But mostly am I grateful for the lives of my friends to whom I have had to say goodbye. I miss you, my brothers. But I thank you, for in the candid sharing of your dying, you provided me with valuable spiritual direction. The only way I can repay you is to pass on your gift. And that is my prayer as I let go of these words. They have a life of their own now. Loving God, if they feed just one soul in need, it will be enough.

Michaelmas 1986
JEF

# CHAPTER 1

## From the Bottom of the Heap

To explore the spiritual meaning of AIDS in the lives of gay people, we need first to talk in general about their spiritual journeys. While the whole of my book *Embracing the Exile*[1] is devoted to that subject, some will not have read it and, what is more, the five years of life since that book's publication have, I hope, led me to some deeper insights. So at the risk of repetition, this chapter will attempt to describe in broad outline the spiritual landscape of gay people's lives.

### *What Does* Spiritual *Mean?*

To begin, it is necessary to be clear about what the word *spiritual* means. It is such a loaded term: people use it to refer to anything from the phantasmagoric mystical experiences of hermits in caves to evangelical-pentecostal-charismatic fervor. Neither of those dramatic human endeavors is what I generally have in mind when I use the word. By *spiritual* I refer to things that are both much more everyday and at the same time much more elusive than either of the just-mentioned extremes.

By *spiritual* I allude to the journey of the soul—not to religion itself but to the drive in humankind that gives rise to religion in the first place. I have in mind the software on the computer of life, not its hardware; the program as it runs, not the data to be input or the machine that processes it or even the printout. By *spiritual* I am referring to that aura around all of our lives that gives what we do meaning, the human striving toward meaning, the search for a sense of belonging.

Writing about things spiritual ultimately must be more aesthetical than logical. We cannot pin spirituality down and study it as if it were a scholarly discipline like theology or history or science. We can only point toward the Holy; we can only trick ourselves or others into the presence of what Rudolf Otto called the numinous; we can only catch glimpses of God's life and power. These are mysteries that evade us in direct proportion to how resolutely we grab for them.

I am going to write about spirituality even though I know most gay people associate it with the Church and, having been alienated from the Church, are immediately suspicious even of the word *spiritual*. But it is precisely *because* most gay people have been alienated by the Church that I *keep* writing about spirituality, because I am convinced that all of us have spiritual needs: the need for grounding, some deep sense of belonging in a cosmic context. And these needs are not being met in contemporary Western society.

The Church has not done well in helping us gay and lesbian people on our spiritual journeys. In its terror of sexuality, it has been singularly put off by those of us whose sexuality, by ontological chance, is remarkable in its differentness. Gay people draw the

Church's attention to a piece of itself it frequently wishes would go away. Yet, I am convinced that Christianity (which is not the same thing as the Church) can help us. I am forced by study and experience to conclude that the spirituality that Jesus embodied and taught—as well as we can know these things through those frustrating, convoluted, muddy media called Holy Scripture and Tradition—speaks to our situation powerfully.

We who are marginalized by society so often feel like "strangers in a strange land," treated hostilely, as we are, by people who are terrified of what we represent to them. And I am persuaded that Jesus, who knew from personal experience exactly how we feel, points us toward spiritual roots where we can find the kind of grounding we need in order to make our lives—in all of their joys and sorrows—meaningful. And, of course, this experience of being alienated is not known uniquely by gay people.

This is the best I can do to demonstrate how I use the word *spiritual*. And I feel I should add immediately that I do not believe Christianity is the *only* spiritual path. While I believe it lifts up some essential pieces of truth that no other world religion professes, there is wisdom to be found in every tradition. Still, Christianity is *mine* and so I will be writing from within that framework, using Christian symbols and metaphors and images and notions. If Christianity is not *your* tradition, you may need to do some translating of what follows. But I have chosen not to try to make my religious language generic, because I believe my words would then come out distant and tortured. And that is the last thing I want since it is from my center to your center that I want to speak.

### Christianity and Homosexuality

Another matter regarding spirituality should be mentioned in a prefatory way. Many people cannot consider homosexuality and Christianity simultaneously without immediately bumping up against those six (or was it seven?) supposedly salient passages of the Hebrew and Christian scriptures that appear to be talking about homosexuality. Those passages will not be dealt with here. I will stop only long enough to cite Robin Scroggs's book *The New Testament and Homosexuality*[2] as the definitive work on this topic. I fully agree with Dr. Scroggs's conclusions (and those of many eminent theologians today) that the passages in the Bible that are often dragged out to flog gay people have absolutely nothing to do with constitutionally gay and lesbian people in mutual, caring relationships. They cannot be used, but are only abused, when quoted to speak to our situation in any way at all.

I am also not planning to spend much time in this chapter reflecting on the Church and its relationship to homosexuality, the issue, or with homosexual people. For that, I recommend John Boswell's excellent book *Christianity, Social Tolerance, and Homosexuality*.[3] Again, I will mention just one striking conclusion of Boswell's research, namely, that more often in the history of the Church than contemporary Christian reactionaries want to be made aware of, we gay and lesbian folk have been *blessed* on our way.

When we have been blessed, we have been enabled

to pass blessing on. During those periods, we have provided Christendom with a disproportionately large number of its most creative, innovative, charismatic and compassionate ministers, priests, bishops, teachers and prophets.

However, the converse needs to be said as well. During those periods when gay people have been cursed on our way (as is the case nowadays), there still have been numerous gay clergy. But out of the covertness that such oppression promotes among gay clergy who must try to be both priest or minister (their true vocation) and gay (their true sexuality) comes much cursedness in the Church. Lonely, isolated gay priests in remote backwaters quietly drinking themselves to death. Gay ministers trying to pastor—by definition an intimate undertaking—but having to leave an enormous piece of their personhood outside the pastoral relationship. Quietly seething congregations who must deal with an evasive gay Father, who is present but never really present. Gay priests or ministers who vote at Church conventions or synods or conferences for the oppression of gay people in order to protect their reputations. There are literally thousands of clergy in such situations in the Church today, leading schizophrenic, anxious lives. If we could only lift up their wholeness, how much blessing the Church would know once again. But before I digress any farther, let us turn to the matter at hand.

### Union with God

Spirituality is about the journey of the soul toward union with God. That is how we Christians have traditionally said it. In the East, the goal of the journey is said to be *atma* or *samadhi* or *satori* or enlightenment or cosmic consciousness. Experientially, I would contend these are the same. But some clarity will be gained, I think, if we Westerners try on the Eastern phraseology for a while.

The Christian notion of union with God has its dangers. On the one hand, it tends to encourage us to anthropomorphize God, to see God in human terms. Which is all right to a point. I have never forgotten a phrase of John MacQuarrie's, that "if God is the All, then God is *at least* personal."[4] But the danger is that by visualizing the deity as a person, we can come to *limit* Her in our minds.

One trap we can fall into at this point is to put God conveniently and comfortably in a box on some altar, or into a wafer or a Holy Book, or to make Him our very own "personal" (read: mine-and-not-yours) savior. Once in this trap, we reduce God (in our minds) to proportions small enough to allow us to deceive ourselves into believing that we have Her under control. We then begin to behave as though we owned God.

The alternate danger inherent in the notion of union with God is that we begin to see this God who is a Being separate from us as *very* separate from us, whose life is not really *in* us at all. Our religion then ceases to be incarnational and we place ourselves in a schizophrenic universe. Either union with God begins to be experienced as an eternally unrealizable hope, or we split ourselves, usually along body-soul lines, trouncing our bodies and yearning for our soul's eventual union with the divine (about which much more will be said in chapter 2). Neither of these paths ultimately will help us on our spiritual journey.

"Cosmic consciousness" may seem like a chilly phrase to Westerners, but it does remind us that God is "the All." To experience God is to experience the oneness of all that is. To know God is to know the universe as a seamless garment. So then, if we Christians want to talk about achieving union with God, we must also want to experience ourselves as connected with all of creation and all of God's creatures. It means we must also come to know the God *within*, experiencing our own inner connectedness and unity.

This kind of spiritual experience leads to an unshakable sense of belonging in our skins and in the universe. And this is the goal of the spiritual journey: a vibrant awareness of the oneness of everything. To love God is to be in love with the universe. This all might be viewed as Idea One of the spiritual path.

### The Spiritual Journey

Idea Two involves the challenge of reaching that kind of consciousness. Spiritual growth is mostly an intuitive process; but we humans tend mostly to know *facts*. Especially in the twentieth century, left to our own devices, we tend to be left-brain, cognitive beings. We yearn to know individual, discreet things. If we combine facts, it is usually in a logical, analytic way. But this does *not* lead to spiritual growth. One cannot proceed rationally into greater spiritual depth. There is no way to *think* our way into the kingdom. It is necessary to leap there.

The process still begins with our human observation of discreet facts. But the intuitive experience is one of glimpsing the connectedness of all things by experiencing the connectedness of many discreet things. And this is true both for things outside of us and inside of us. Spiritual growth is more of the nature of proceeding from hunch to hunch than from conclusion to conclusion.

Now, it is in the *interior* universe that we who are gay most often get stuck in our souls' journeyings. So we will need to take a closer look at why this is.

We come to know our inner wholeness by becoming increasingly acquainted with the marvelous, complex web that each of us is. To know myself as a "child of God" is to know my inner unity, to know in the depths of my soul that I am one as God is one. Repeated glimpses of this connectedness lead to an intuitive knowing that I am created in the image of God, the One who is the unity of everything.

From my vantage point, this voyage toward knowing the All within us is the beginning of the spiritual journey. Moreover, it is the single most important task any of us could be about. In this frighteningly fragmented world, to spend time and energy coming to know wholeness cannot be construed as a luxury; it simply must have first priority. Until we experience our inner unity, we will never be able to externalize it. Conversely, to the extent that we know ourselves as splintered, we will continue to create chaos in the world about us.

A dramatic externalized international example of

the shallowness of our sense of connectedness is what we do societally with the distribution of food in the world. Every day, some 95,000 of God's children—our brothers and sisters—starve to death.[5] Lest that be glossed over as a statistic, I would like you to pause for a moment and try to visualize 95,000 emaciated, dead bodies. (Images of corpses stacked in Nazi concentration camps would approximate the scene.) Bodies of men, women, and children. Pause again and try to grasp for a moment the physical excruciation that just one of those 95,000 people went through in the process of dying. And then sit for a while longer and contemplate that this is a *daily* routine.

In contrast, consider that more than 220,000 United States citizens die each year from cardiovascular disease, caused mostly by obesity and the eating of over-rich foods. Sixty-three percent of us are clinically overweight.[6] And in order to deal with an economy troubled by food surpluses, the U.S. government pays farmers millions of dollars annually *not* to grow grain.

In spite of the grotesque inequity exposed by these publicly available statistics, 96 percent of United States citizens profess to be Christian[7] and would undoubtedly claim that they espouse such values as justice and care for the poor, the homeless, and the hungry.

Now clearly, there is no way an entire population could tolerate the scathing self-indictment that a grasp of this combination of facts must prompt unless there were a generalized and profound lack of consciousness. Only a severe form of spiritual fragmentation can explain how we live with these horrible realities.

The point here is that this international dilemma

begins in each of our souls. And until we know our inner cohesiveness, we will continue to create the splintered, cruel world in whose perpetuation we all participate.

We know our inner wholeness more or less. Mostly less. When we experience that lack of wholeness, we sometimes say of ourselves that we are "broken," or "damaged," or "sick," or "sinful." I believe these are all inaccurate and unhelpful ways of describing that experience. Rather than helping us grow, they serve only to reinforce our already split consciousnesses.

When we refer to ourselves as "broken" or "damaged," we are usually really describing pieces of ourselves that do not *feel* connected, parts of us that we reject or repress or quarantine. We are not *actually* broken; the God in whom I believe does not make "seconds." We only *think* we are broken. What we call brokenness, then, is only a matter of not knowing wholeness.

For gay people, the biggest piece of us that seems not to fit is our sexuality. We have been carefully taught. It is not necessarily that we out-and-out reject our gayness; it is more often a matter of our not believing that it is part of our wholeness. We who are gay so often cordon our sexuality off from the rest of who we are, thereby compartmentalizing our selves through a frightening process of practiced splitting.[8]

We have had lots of help. Society, for instance, would generally prefer us split, and actively thwarts our attempts at behaving in a more integrated manner. And how many gay institutions (bars, baths) have continued to support the dichotomy—our sexual selves in one social sphere and the rest of us in another. For the great good the gay liberation movement has accomplished, its major failing has been this: it has assumed that all we had to do was lift up the gay and we would be free. How often this has degenerated into liberation's meaning no more than the ability to indulge any appetite with impunity. Of course, this is not liberation at all, as we have learned the hard way. (I am reminded of the Kris Kristofferson lyric, "Freedom's just another word for nothin' left to lose . . . ") This approach leaves our cleft souls as bifurcated as ever, as a story will illustrate.

I have a friend named Jim. He is an Episcopal priest who used to live in New York City. Jim used to observe a weekly ritual of donning his leather and spending Saturday night at the Mineshaft (which, in case you are unfamiliar with the gay subculture, was probably the sleaziest gay bar in New York, now closed, where one could get any variety of sex in any quantity one wanted). Then, Sunday morning early, Jim would stumble home, change into his clericals and go assist at Solemn High Mass at one of our most high-church institutions (and in case you are unacquainted with Episcopal lore, "high-church" refers to a highly liturgical establishment where one can virtually glut oneself on ritual and choke oneself on incense every Sunday of the year).

So every week for Jim it was Saturday night in leather at the Mineshaft and Sunday morning in brocade at High Mass. And you had better believe that he would never have thought of identifying himself as a priest at the Mineshaft nor, in a straightforward way, owned his gayness at church.

Jim always insisted he was both a liberated gay man and a devout Christian. His compulsive pursuit of each of these identities, seeking the most excessive institutional expression in each sphere, always spoke to me of his yearning to affirm them both as one, and his thinking that this was the way to do it. But mostly what I experienced in Jim was the fissure in his consciousness attested to by the incredible gulf between those two aspects of his life. During that whole part of his journey, he never recognized the rift. He did not see that those two inextricable parts of who he was were connected—*really* connected. By how he lived his life, Jim clearly did not believe that his sexuality comprised part of the God-given wholeness that he was. And in that splitting of his head, I do not believe Jim was unique in the gay community. I think he was typical. Nor do I think things have changed much. (By the way, Jim is very different now, although I frankly think he gave up his old habits more out of sheer exhaustion than spiritual enlightenment. The Lord works in mysterious ways.)

So the question of how to get there most often becomes: How do we put these pieces together in our heads? How do we go about healing our broken view of ourselves? Well, to begin with, it is hard. We have been carefully *taught* that our sexuality does not fit. This notion of fragmentation is not one with which we were born; it was ingrained in us and reinforced for us in both subtle and obvious ways. So I would be lying if I said there is not hard work involved. But it is a strange kind of hard work.

The West has little to offer us on this part of the

journey. Christianity has largely lost its spiritual roots. We have forgotten that to know God, one must begin by *shutting up*. We have no equivalent of the exquisitely developed Eastern disciplines that encourage silence and teach people how to use solitude fruitfully.[9] (The only close approximation of this in Christendom are the Ignatian *Spiritual Exercises*, which, in my estimation, are still primitive in comparison with the spiritual practices of, say, Zen Buddhism or Hinduism.) As it is, in most Christian churches—tell me if this is not true—if there are thirty contiguous seconds of silence during Sunday morning worship, everyone assumes the organist has screwed up.

I mention all of this only to drive home the essential truth about the spiritual path: the journey begins by quieting one's insides, making room, leaving time to hear and to notice. There is no magic about this. The practice of spiritual growth has as its core the practice of silence. With no further direction at all, if one spent thirty minutes a day just sitting, one would be halfway home. I cannot emphasize enough the simple, but easily skipped over, importance of this truth.

The old Christian "spiritual disciplines" revolving around penance, devotions, discursive (that is, thought-full) meditations, examinations of conscience leading to the practice of self-loathing, self-denial, and a rejection of this world in favor of some disembodied spiritual state or some future pie-in-the-sky heaven all reflect notions that are, in my opinion, unrelated to what Jesus came preaching. They are certainly not supported by what He Himself did. As will be discussed more fully in chapter 2, I am persuaded that the only healthy thing we can do with most of those ill-balanced approaches to Christian spirituality is to leave them behind. And lest I be misunderstood, I really am quite explicitly contending that the spirituality espoused by most of the church fathers, from Origen until the Reformation, in its imbalance was thoroughly detrimental to spiritual growth.

What we need to do to enable spiritual growth is what Jesus did. He spent goodly amounts of time *alone*. What is more, He lived His life with an almost (for us) incomprehensible awareness of the connectedness of everything both within Him and around Him. And finally, with this cosmic awareness, He acted, one might say, in the very center of His life. There was a cohesiveness about all that Jesus did, and a simplicity. He merely did what each moment required, no more, no less. The firsthand writings about Him seem to describe a man who was ultimately calm, centered, and clear, despite the turmoil surrounding Him. He knew His place in the universe; He knew what He needed to be about.

Here again, the East gives us nonloaded language to express these notions. A guru might say that spiritual deepening involves a journey toward the unselfconscious living of life as it unfolds rather than toward a willful determination to *make it happen*. The spiritual path is about simple unity. It is the antithesis of empire-building, with all of its complexities and convolutions and power struggles. It is about living ever more profoundly in this moment, sensing the truth in the Zen epithet that claims, "All that is, is now." It leads to diminishing the amount of energy we spend seething or gloating over past victories or defeats. It makes future dangers or conquests seem unimportant. To say this psychologically, spiritual growth leads toward the disenfranchisement of our power-hungry egos, which are constantly trying to fix, name, control, categorize, and insure all of our experience.[10]

Unlike much pop psychology, the spiritual journey is not interested in helping us transform our negative self-images into positive ones. Have you noticed how someone's preoccupation with self-hate can yield almost miraculously to popular "personal power" experiences only to be replaced by something just shy of megalomania? You see, self-hate and self-aggrandizement are equally binding; one is no improvement over the other. The self remains our preoccupation either way, blinding us from perceiving reality in all of its enormity.

And so, the hard work I am talking about is not of the nature of something that you do, as in "If I sit in a lotus position two hours a day for ten years . . . " or "If I say a rosary every day . . . " or "If I do an Ignatian retreat . . . " or "If I go to a yoga class every week . . . then, *then*, THEN I will get spiritually deeper." It will not work. (Although I would heartily encourage you to try it if you must, at least until you reach a point of exasperation.) This learning is much more a matter of *not* doing, or maybe of *not* not doing—of letting be, or letting go. Barry Stevens captured the notion in the title of her book, *Don't Push the River*.[11] You cannot try to stop pushing the river (Could you have pushed it anyway?); you can only just stop pushing the river. In the same way, you cannot achieve spiritual depth by exerting effort, but only by letting things be.

By the way, I am not advocating passivity or quietism or navel contemplation in any of this. I am often accused of that, especially by activists of one stripe or another. We are not called to be dumb, all-yielding sheep who should lie down and die in the face of oppression. No. Responding to the moment means responding to what goes on *inside* of us as well as around us. Quite in contrast to acquiescence, I am talking about being acutely present to the moment, acutely aware of what is going on in *both* spheres and then doing what the moment requires. And that response may mean being quite animated in one way or another. The difference being addressed here is more a matter of whether an activity is ego-driven or whether it proceeds uncoerced from our spiritual center.

In sum, I am saying that to undertake the spiritual journey, we need to find some method that works for us so that we can practice becoming quiet inside. Only this will lead to healing the broken view we hold of ourselves. And, of course, this is not something that one ever does once and for all; it is a lifetime pursuit.

Unfortunately, groups or churches or institutions that can help us on this journey are few and far between. But the major components of the discipline are not esoteric. They involve making time to be silent and, in that silence, trying to experience 'all that is' in its broadest possible terms. At least some Quaker meetings are committed to engendering silence as the cornerstone of the spiritual journey. And a few other Christian organizations (like the Shalem Institute for

Spiritual Formation in Washington, D.C.) have arisen explicitly to foster meditative practice and to train bona fide spiritual directors. But many people have made the journey in total isolation, although certainly, support from fellow travelers is of enormous help and comfort.

This, then, constitutes Idea Two, the "how to" of the spiritual path.

### A Digression

We probably should digress here so that you can ask a couple of the kinds of questions most people ask at this point, like 'Why bother?' and 'Why go through all of this?' They are fair questions. Most people would never touch any of this stuff with a fork. How do they manage? Are they happy?

In place of spiritual deepening, our society offers us a very elaborate and attractive myth, a collective societal ruse that begins with a premise: that we are, indeed, autonomously powerful. That *we* are God, that *I* am the All. This has been codified in the "personal power" movement, whose cornerstone epithet might be phrased this way: "I can get anything I want; if I'm not getting it, I'm doing it wrong."

I will admit my prejudice. I believe this is acquired insanity: it is the ego gone wild. It is the ego enthroned. Rather than being empowered, we demand to be in power. Unsatisfied with being creatures, we determine to be Creators. This myth has brought us face-to-face with the ever-present terror of nuclear disaster; it has institutionalized mass starvation; it has spawned every possible form of political exploitation; and it has created a culture of unbridled narcissism.[12] Other than that, it has a great deal to commend it.

Well, in fact, the myth does have one payoff, which is why it is so popular. Pretending that we are God holds anxiety at bay. The ego (the ME, in actual Freudian terms) is a strange, enigmatic, and tenacious beast. I need ME to survive and yet ME can be my own worst enemy. To surrender, to let go, to just *be*—as the spiritual path requires—*is* frightening. There is initially a sense of being out of control. The ME sends up a red flag saying, "This will lead to disaster!" So even though the societal myth is a fake, a fraud, our acting as though we were autonomous and self-determining helps quell the fear that comes from realizing the truth: that in the face of the All, we are virtually powerless.

In the face of a little fragile bug named HIV, in the face of a Colombian earthquake, in the face of a terrorist attack, in the face of an awesome universe whose very dimensions we cannot fathom, how powerful are we? These are the sobering facts and the myth helps keep all of this disturbing reality out of sight and, we hope, out of mind. And except when the set develops cracks and the terror breaks through, most people prefer to live with the deception.

What does the spiritual path offer instead? A powerful sense of being grounded in this moment, in this body, in this room, in this universe. A feeling of being plugged in, empowered, fully alive. Ultimately, a sense of inner peacefulness and inner cohesiveness and imperturbability that can transcend the most painful of situations and make the joyful ones ecstatic. That is the payoff. And I cannot speak for you, but in these days of "future shock," I could do with some of that. But it comes at a cost. The price one must pay for this equanimity is living with the angst of our infinitesimalness. It is a price most people apparently are unwilling to pay.

### The Gay Dilemma

Idea Three. Those of us who are gay or lesbian face a special dilemma and opportunity in the course of our spiritual journeys. For the most part, we who are gay—especially if we are candid about our sexuality—are excluded from the societal myth presented a moment ago. The power structures, the sanctions, and the ego-pacifying outlets that are afforded most people are denied us. We face the same anxiety everyone else faces about being powerless—our egos are just as eager to try to convince us of our godlike autonomy—but we are intentionally, often forcefully, shut out from those mythic societal constructs that might give us the same false but convenient sense of security other people get to take advantage of. We are, if you will, exiled, forced to the outskirts of the great mythic promised land society has to offer.

I will digress one more time here to defend my perception of the ongoing nature of this oppression. I hear and read a good deal of rhetoric in gay circles that disagrees with this point of view. There is a not uncommon belief that gay people in the 1980s are almost fully liberated. There is simply no foundation for this belief.

First, I cite a 1983 *Psychology Today*[13] poll in which 70 percent of the respondents said they felt gay people should not teach school, 50 percent opposed our being physicians, and 30 percent (!) contended we were unfit to be sales clerks. And, since *Psychology Today*'s readership is probably heavily weighted with upper-middle-class Caucasian Americans, the likelihood is that a more representative cross-section of the United States would reflect even more oppressive views.

The pretext of AIDS to justify blatant oppression of gay people and the concomitant rise in violence against us in the past three years is further evidence of deep-seated ongoing homophobia.

And finally, we must be very careful not to generalize from the urban sociological situation to all of the United States. While gay people in urban areas may be able to live quite comfortably these days (unless they aspire to be professionals), it is still a very frightening thing to be gay or lesbian in rural or even small-town America.

In the face of exclusion from this myth—in the face of this exile—most gay people, being human, try to escape. Some of the ways we choose to try to avoid the pain are very self-destructive. In the gay community, alcoholism is 300 percent higher than in society as a whole. Suicide is four times as frequent.[14] The wild, woolly, and often kinky sexual world that the gay subculture in the past has offered (and that AIDS has largely precluded) was, for some, another way to loosen one's brains and obliterate the pain.

Then again, some of us try to gain reentry into the

myth, either by guile (the closet) or by force (militancy). We want power. We want equality. Acceptance. Sanctions. Restitution. What we *want* is a piece of the action. We want a piece of that myth. And who knows? If we keep pushing, we may eventually get it. As they have with blacks and to a lesser extent women, the White Heterosexual Male Supremacist Club that works hard to keep us on the fringes may eventually tire of the game and say, "Oh, what the hell, why not let them build a few houses of cards of their own?"

But a striking question I would like us to ask ourselves in the interim—and I suspect the interim will continue for some time—is this: Do we want that myth? Do we really want it? And therein, I think, is both the irony . . . and the opportunity of our predicament. Excluded from a myth that might give us a false sense of security, we who are gay are confronted with the genuine, if stark and sometimes painful, truth of who we are in all of our creatureliness. Being exiled puts us intimately in touch with our powerlessness, it is true, but precisely because we are confronted with that awareness, we are also given the opportunity of spiritual empowerment. We are, if we will only let go, thrust down to our spiritual roots.

Most often, we cry, "Why me?" And if that is your response, I cannot fault you. We did not choose to be here. And it is not fair. But the fact is, it is where we find ourselves when we are truly being who we are, living in the center of our lives, taking what this moment offers, and doing what this moment requires. It seems as though the fringes are the place from which we are called to share our gifts. It is precisely from the bottom of the societal heap that we seem called to spread the Good News.

I have come to experience that position as a very powerful place to be. And I offer a story in hopes that you might glimpse its power, too.

### The Opportunity

Ten years ago, a man named Wayne and I were members of a radical inner-city Episcopal parish in Washington, D.C., called the Church of St. Stephen and the Incarnation. In the sixties, St. Stephen's was where, after Dr. Martin Luther King, Jr.'s death, Rap Brown preached while Washington burned one block away. It was where, eleven years ago, four women were "irregularly" ordained to the Episcopal priesthood. It was the parish whose rector, William Wendt, was tried and found guilty by an ecclesiastical court for allowing one of those ordained women to celebrate the Eucharist. It has been one of the most avant-garde places of liturgical renewal in the Church. And it was where, in 1976, Wayne and I were encouraged by the rector and congregation to celebrate the sanctity of our relationship in a service of Holy Union.

Needless to say, ten years ago that was a cheeky and foolish thing to do. I cannot begin to relate in a few paragraphs the turmoil, the beauty, but most of all the pain that surrounded the whole event. While most of the parish was firmly behind us, there emerged a substantial minority of older, conservative Episcopalians who were not amused. Blacks were fine, women priests were fine, crazy liturgies were fine, but gay unions were past their limit. They caused quite a ruckus. Several families left the parish; the rest simply shunned Wayne and me from that time on. Which hurt. And it was the response of virtually every parishioner aged fifty to sixty except one. We shall name her Mary MacLean Selcik; it is her story I want to tell.

Mary was a proper Scottish lady in her sixties who had married young. She had not had a happy life. Her marriage had failed, a hard thing for a proper Scottish lady to take. One of her sons was psychotic, in and out of institutions. Her career at the U.S. State Department had been an uphill struggle, mostly because Mary's sense of justice would not allow her to remain silent in the face of the then-rampant inequity being doled out to her and her black and female co-workers.

She always seemed to me a courageous but despairing person. A woman of great dignity . . . and sadness. A woman who blamed herself for everything that went badly in her life. A woman who carried around enormous guilt.

I suppose it was Mary's innate sense of justice that would not allow her to dismiss Wayne and me as her peers had done. Every Sunday morning, at the passing of the peace, as the rest of her age-group made big circles around me, she would come directly up, firmly grasp my hand with both of hers, look me right in the eye, smile warmly, and say, "Good morning, my dear."

About a year later, Mary disappeared from St. Stephen's. It was such a frenetic place that I failed to notice her absence for a while. But when I finally inquired about her, I was told confidentially that Mary had lung cancer and was dying. Her way of coping with this final failure (as she apparently saw it) was to leave St. Stephen's and Washington and to remove herself to a rural Virginia town where she planned on dying alone. The parishioner who told me this added that I was not supposed to know it and that I must not try to contact her.

Well, I tried to honor her request, but I couldn't. I just couldn't. She had meant much to me. So eventually, I sleuthed out her address and wrote. I told her how much I had valued her having stood by Wayne and me the year before when we were going through hard times. I told her how much I wanted to reciprocate now that hard times had befallen her. I offered to come visit, run errands, read to her, whatever.

Four months passed. No response. I assumed I had indeed gaffed by writing. I tried to forget about it. Then one day, Mary's letter arrived. She wrote that she had been in the hospital and really had been unable to write. She told me how beautiful my letter had seemed to her. She told me that Bill Wendt had been helping her grieve her impending death. And finally, she wrote that she would be moving back to Washington and would like nothing better than for us to have some time together to sit and talk, as she wrote, "of shoes and ships and sealing wax, of cabbages and kings."

She returned to Washington about a month later, but before we could manage even one get-together, Mary MacLean Selcik died. I was bereft, left with a strong sense of incompletion both with her and about her in terms of how unsettled she had seemed to the end. The night after she died, Bill Wendt, who had been at her deathbed, and I were officiating at the

Eucharist. As we were taking off our vestments in the sacristy after the service, I mused to Bill that it seemed Mary had never made it to a peaceful place; that she seemed to have *died* with her courageous despair; dignified, but sad and guilt-ridden to the end.

"No," Bill said, matter-of-factly. "No, she made it. And it all had to do with the letter you sent her." I couldn't imagine what he meant; I had long since forgotten the letter. "The night before she died," Bill went on, "with her family around her, Mary pulled that letter from the drawer of her nightstand. She passed it around the room and made every single one of her family from oldest to youngest read it. And then she announced calmly and surely and peacefully, "That young man has given me a most wonderful gift. By his love, he has shown me that many kinds of people can be Christian . . ." And she added through her tears, ". . . even me. Even me."

Regardless of what Holy Orders I may ever be permitted to take, I will always view that day as my commissioning, my ordination. Because I came to know in that event that the most powerful place from which to renew the face of the earth is the bottom of the heap.

I often think of the motley crew of gay and lesbian Christian refugees I hang out with as a remnant, as our Jewish forebears in the desert were a remnant. Banished from Egypt with no sure home to go to, with no comfortable societal myth to hide behind, they too were thrust down to their spiritual roots. And in that desolate place, they glimpsed in an incredibly powerful way the unity of God. "Hear, O Israel, the LORD is our God. The LORD alone" (Deut. 6:4).

It was a revelation that changed the face of history. As Jesus—a remnant of one—irrevocably altered the course of history. Jesus, "despised and rejected of men" whose exile led Him to such spiritual depth and to such powerful loving that those of us who are Christians say He *was* the All.

The alternative to trying to force our way back into the myth is to embrace our exile. Not passively. Not with resignation. But with vigor and passion. Drinking deeply from the cup we have been passed as an oppressed people, seeing it as an opportunity both for profound spiritual deepening and for being empowered to do some very holy work in an especially potent way.

And what is that work? Oh, just to love. And in our case, frequently enough, to love *anyway*. To give when nobody wants your gifts. To be present when many would like us to go away. To speak our pain when most people would rather ignore it. We are called to *be*. To be fully who we are. In the moment. In the world. That is loving.

There will be old hurts to let go of and some dreams for the future as well. We will have to forego many of the fake comforts of being in society's good graces. Most of us will never get to be yuppies. But in that wilderness that seems to be our portion and cup, I am convinced we will touch and be touched by God very powerfully.

If the lives of our Jewish forebears, or of Jesus, the Christ, or of so many of the holy men and women we meet in history or on the street who have suffered for justice's sake are any indication, loving in the face of oppression is a show-stopper. Doing justice with all your guts when what the world has for you mostly is contempt speaks God's love very potently. It also confuses the hell out of people. But of greatest importance, it seems to renew the face of the earth.

I believe this is the mission to which we are called, we who are gay men and lesbian women committed to affirming our sexual-spiritual wholeness. But it will take striking our spiritual roots very deep. Deep into the moment. Deep into the cosmos. Deep into the bosom of God.

## Coda

Before moving on, an important acknowledgment must be made. The spiritual journey, dilemma, and opportunity just described are by no means the exclusive property of the gay community. We are *all* in one way or another, in exile. We are all "not home." That is the plight of us creatures in this post-Resurrection, pre-Parousia situation. Whether one is black or a woman, divorced, handicapped, damaged from childhood abuse, a teenager, or a person with AIDS (no matter how one contracted it), we have all tasted the abyss. I have written this chapter from the poignant exile of being gay because it is what I know best. But we are all invited to drink this cup in all of its bitter-sweetness. It is the quintessence of being human.

In the next chapter, we will examine what the Church and Western civilization bring to the AIDS crisis—the worldview they presume in coming to grips with it. And then in chapter 3, we will turn to the spiritual meaning of AIDS itself.

# CHAPTER 2

# Disembodiment:
# The Orthodox Heresy

Why has AIDS stirred up such strong feelings? More to the point, why has Western civilization been so confronted by this *particular* disease? And why has there been so much renewed violence against gay people since AIDS began spreading in the Western hemisphere? These questions point to the need for deeper examination of society's assumptions about AIDS and death and homosexuality.

An answer to these queries cannot have only to do with fear of exposure to a deadly virus. Since medical authorities have repeatedly made clear that AIDS cannot be communicated through casual contact, the reaction we are witnessing must come from someplace else, someplace deeper, someplace in people's souls that is patently not rational.

AIDS has, in fact, opened a Pandora's box of unfinished spiritual business. And we will find no answers to the questions just posed unless we go back and explore where the spiritual accounts were left unbalanced.

It is my contention that we will find the roots of our dilemma firmly anchored at the doorstep of Holy Mother Church. The Church's historic attitude toward creation, mortality, sensuousness,[1] sex, and bodies insinuated itself almost from its inception into the fabric of Western civilization. It continues to do so. And while this worldview has affected all aspects of our lives, some facets of it have had serious consequences for how American society is now responding to AIDS. It is these facets that we will investigate.

### Heresy Defined

The subtitle of this chapter, "The Orthodox Heresy," fairly summarizes my view of this strand of the Church's history. I am going to make what may seem like an outrageous assertion, namely that for almost two thousand years—from the time Jesus preached until today—the Church has almost exclusively lifted up only half of the truth Jesus taught in one crucial area of reality. And while it may sound shocking to some, I am going to define this imbalance as heresy. It is, then, my view that the Christian Church has lived in heresy for almost all of its history. This, of course, demands substantiation. I want to disclaim at the outset that I am following in the footsteps of Adolf Harnack, the historical theologian of the early twentieth century, who claimed that, in adopting Greek philosophy, from Paul until the present, the Church got it all wrong. But I am contending that in one critical area, it has got things *half* wrong.)

The word *heresy* derives from the Greek word meaning to grasp or seize. It does not so much connote affirming something that is totally erroneous as it refers to seizing upon only *part* of some truth. Classic examples of this are most of the christological heresies of the early Church. These all basically had to do with some group's or individual's inability to live with the paradox of Jesus' full divinity and full humanity. To achieve psychological relief, they lifted up too high or too exclusively one or the other. It was not that they were wrong; it was that they were only half right.

Now I would propose a theory about heresy. It is this: *heresy* is an institutional word, a word that establishments get to use. Organizations like the Church call heretical those minority positions that they find threatening.

But I would contend that the Church simply cannot do without its heretics because, in most instances, these dissidents have arisen in the Church to correct an imbalance (heresy) that already exists in the Church. For example, it seems clear that the Reformation was a necessary corrective in the course of the Church's unfolding. The Reformers lifted up (albeit with a vengeance) faith and the Word in a Church that had lapsed into rampant works-ism and superstitious "liturgiolatry."

All of this is to prepare the way for contending that the Church has, technically, been in heresy from its beginning in its attitude, piety, and practice concerning bodies and souls. It has taken one road through this country; it has left the other unexplored. Moreover, it has held "the road not taken" largely in contempt for almost two thousand years, basically unchallenged until the Reformation, only slightly mitigated until Vatican II, and subliminally in force even into the present in many ways. These philosophical underpinnings have affected every aspect of Western civilization.

The dilemma that the Church and society now face and that they conceptualize in terms like "a crisis of sexual ethics" or "a culture of narcissism" or "the problem of sexuality" really stems from the corner into which they have consistently painted themselves on matters like bodies, physicality, sensuality, and worldliness. And in order to get out of that corner (which is crucial if we are ever to create spiritual life out of the AIDS crisis), we will need to retrace our steps. This will, naturally, require walking through a sticky mess.

## The Historical Backdrop

Christianity arose during a very unstable period in the history of Israel. This is not to say that either the people, Israel, or the land of Canaan had ever been peaceful for long. The tribe or tribes who became identified as Israelites had come into the land about two thousand years before Jesus' birth. At least some of them apparently migrated to Egypt during a famine, stayed there a long time, escaped during a period of persecution, wandered in the desert for another long time, reentered Canaan some twelve hundred years before Jesus was born, took over the area in some way, solidified themselves into a theocratic nation, were conquered by Babylon and Persia, and largely carried off into captivity about seven hundred years before Jesus lived. About fifty years later, some Israelites returned to Canaan; most never did. And except for a brief period, the Jewish people would not know political autonomy again until 1948.

Upon the fall of the Persian Empire, Israel was taken by Alexander the Great of Greece (333 B.C.), then by the Ptolemies (culturally Greek), then by the Seleucids (culturally Greek again) and then, just sixty years before Jesus was born, by Rome, under whose rule Judea chafed while Jesus lived on earth.

Jesus was a Jew and never thought of himself as anything else. One will not find any scriptures in which Jesus walks up to someone and says, "Hello, I am Jesus of Nazareth, the founder of Christianity." Jesus was a Jew. But he was a Jew in a land ruled by the Roman Empire, a land in which there were many non-Jews, a land in which many cities had no Jewish population at all, a land that had been greatly affected by Hellenism for over three hundred years.

Now all of this historical information may seem far afield from the Church's attitude toward bodies and the world and sensuality. But it is important to understand this historical backdrop to demonstrate how circumscribed and politically impotent Judaism and the Jewish people were in Judea by the time Jesus was born. By that period Judea in no way provided a pervasive Jewish environment; rather, it provided a predominantly Greco-Roman context in which scattered pockets of Judaism existed. There was, for instance, as thoroughgoing a Greek institution as a gymnasium in the middle of Jerusalem. This is the culture into which Jesus and Christianity were born.

While Greek and Roman philosphy may not have been studied by most people in those days (any more than philosophy is studied by most people in the United States today), Hellenism was in the air. It pervaded the culture, just as a Christian ethic and worldview permeate United States culture, even though we are not, strictly speaking, a Christian nation.

Aramaic and Greek were the languages of the realm. Hebrew was falling rapidly into disuse. By two hundred years before Jesus' birth, so few Jews could read Hebrew that the Hebrew Bible (in traditional Christian terms, the Old Testament) had to be rendered by a group of rabbis into Greek (the translation known today as the Septuagint).

To show how far hellenization had gone in Jerusalem itself, we need only look at the Maccabean revolt. While precipitated by the persecution of Antiochus Epiphanes, what we frequently forget about that uprising is that it was also in part a kind of civil war. On one side were hellenized Jews in Jerusalem, who were perfectly happy to give up circumcision and monotheism and the Levitical law and install Zeus in the temple. On the other side were those Jews who would settle for nothing less than the pure religion of Moses.

In sum, Christianity was born into a Greek world. And that had enormous consequences. While it began as a mutation of Judaism, as Christianity expanded and increasingly rejected its Jewish roots, it came quickly and naturally under the influence of Hellenistic philosophy and theology.

This influence in Christianity's earliest days can be demonstrated by comparing the Hebrew and Christian Scriptures. There are only vague hints of Greek influence in the Hebrew books of the Bible, and even then,

only in the later writings. In contrast, Greek philosophical language and concepts are commonplace in
the New Testament.

But hellenization did not stop at the earliest days.
Greek and Roman thought continued to influence the
Church's development through all of its formative
centuries. Neo-Platonism played an especially key
role; Stoicism a lesser but significant one.

There is no possible way to trace the history of this
relationship in a few pages. Nor can one briefly describe how the insinuation of Greek philosophy into
Christianity was interwoven with other forces affecting the Church's emerging theology, piety, and practice. For example, the early persecution of the
Church, its becoming the state religion, its rapid
growth, and the later disintegration of the Roman Empire comprise an enormous and complex historical
web. However, something can be said in a general
way about the main features of Greek thought as relates to sexuality and how they found their way into
the Church. We can also explore a bit what form these
features took in their new environment.

### The Greek View

The early Christian Church was much taken with
the Greek philosophical notion of human beings existing in two dimensions, body and soul. This concept existed (and may well have originated) elsewhere in the
Near East, but the Church knew it primarily as a Greek
concept and from it drew some unique implications.

If your reaction to this model of humanity as

composed of bodies and souls is that it seems self-evident, it is only because the model has permeated Western civilization for over two thousand years. Many people in the world, both then and now, recognize no such distinction. More specifically, thinking of oneself as a soul who happens to have a body would have seemed ludicrous to most Jews at the time of Jesus. The same would be true of most Jews today.

In this Greek universe, there were two realms, the mortal and the immortal, corresponding to the body and the soul, respectively. But to grasp this in any kind of authentic Greek way, we must understand that these were extremely abstract—nay, esoteric—notions. We must think of them more in terms of spheres than duration. The immortal was the sphere of Being of highest distinction. The gods were immmortal. The human soul was immortal. Beauty and truth were immortal. Associated with immortality were such attributes as absoluteness, rationality, unchangeability, indivisibility, imperturbability, invisibility, and self-sufficiency.

Note that immortality in these terms could *not* be reduced to some flat, linear concept of life after death. That was not its core meaning at all. Rather, immortality referred to a dimension of life that transcended time and space (and that could be experienced *now*).

The mortal, in contrast, had associated with it that which was embodied (corporeal, fleshly), visible, changeable, divisible, filled with passion, and often nonrational (that is, spontaneous).

While this duality as well as the attributes associated

with each realm were assumed by virtually all Greek and Roman philosophers, and the interrelationship between the two and the attitude toward each sphere of existence varied considerably from philosophical school to philosophical school and from age to age. Some accepted the duality as blessed and the two elements as good and complementary. Others exalted the body to the denigration of the soul. Still others came to extol the soul and disdain the body. And of course, as with any philosophy, there were broad spectra of emphasis and subtle nuances of difference in all of these cases.

But it was the latter philosophical strain—the exaltation of souls and the denigration of bodies—that the Christian Church took up in a strikingly untempered way.

### The Jewish View

It is important to note that the Jewish view of reality was radically different from this. First, as we have said, a body-soul dualism was foreign to the Jewish universe. Now it is true that as Jews became hellenized during this period, numbers of them began trying to incorporate Greek philosophical notions into their theology. But in terms of classic Judaism—Judaism as reflected in the Hebrew Scriptures—a human being was whole. There was no perceived divisibility of one's ontology, of one's being. A person was a person.

Perhaps the clearest evidence for this is provided by the Hebrew word for spirit, *ruach*. This is the word used in the first chapter of Genesis, in the sentence that says, " . . . the *ruach* of God moved over the face of the waters." Here it has often been translated as "the Spirit of God . . . " But the word also means just plain old breath (or wind). God enspirits us, breathes air into us. In this Jewish context, spirit is not a separate component of human beings; it is the breath of life in us. In Ecclesiastes, for instance, Qoheleth writes that "God takes back our *ruach* and we die." This only means that God takes the breath out of us; there is no allusion here to our "spirit" being taken "up to heaven" as many Christian commentators have assumed.

Another distinct difference in Hebrew philosophy when contrasted with hellenized Christian philosophy is that there is no comparable Jewish notion for the immortality of human beings. Since there was no body-soul duality, there clearly was no room for "the immortality of the soul." People lived, people died. When you died, your children continued your line, which is how you "survived." But the dead were seen to be either consigned to nothingness, which is what most of the Hebrew scriptures assume, or sent to a murky place called Sheol, which is a world of shades, never clearly defined, but certainly not an abode of glorious everlasting life (as Christians came to define heaven).

Even in late Judaism, allusions to resurrection refer not to any idea of immortal life, but to the actual resurrection of embodied people who were quite dead and gone, not souls freed from bodies, not even Paul's refined concept of some new "glorified" bodies. When Daniel talks about resurrection, he means raised-up whole human beings.

Another distinguishing feature of Judaism's view of life is that, since there was virtually no eschatology, God's blessing was to be known now, in this life in all of its worldliness. Judaism was and is an incredibly incarnational religion. One knows God's love and favor by one's health and happiness and comfort and joy and children and flocks and a beautiful wife or handsome husband and impassioned love and good food and wine. To be quintessentially Jewish was and is to have an insatiable appetite for life. "Eat heartily and drink your wine lustily" wrote the author of Ecclesiastes. "To life! To life! L'chaim!" wrote Sheldon Harnack in *The Fiddler on the Roof*.

Finally (and this bit of Hebrew philosophy is important in terms of seeing what happened in Christianity), the Jewish idea of time was also much simpler than the Greek. While the Greek could envision dimensions of being, for the Jew life was a one-dimensional, linear affair. It began at birth; it ended at death. And in between, it was all of a piece, lived on one plane.

### Early Church Hellenization

Well, what happened? As Christianity pulled away from its Jewish roots (abetted, of course, by the Orthodox Jewish rejection and persecution of Christian Judaism), it came increasingly to use Judaism as a foil. In defining itself, Christianity quickly assumed a defensive posture toward its own heritage. To be

Christian was to be *not* Jewish. And, as we shall see, to define oneself *against* someone or something is ultimately an impoverishing act.

In place of its original conception in the Jewish worldview, from the earliest church fathers on, the soul was radically elevated to a position of blessedness and godliness, and the attributes of immortality were deemed the only ones worthy to be striven for. To have achieved them was to have achieved sainthood, the closest any mortal could get to human perfection.

Conversely, the body came quickly to be seen as the prison that kept the soul from being free. The attributes descriptively and (often) nonjudgmentally associated with mortality by early Greek philosophers became bywords of human failure and sinfulness to the early Church.

Passion, irrationality, desire, changeablity, and fleshliness came to be viewed as unholy. This meant that enjoyment of sensual pleasure (taste or sight, touch or sound, food or wine, or sex); or any kind of spontaneity (as might be expressed in dance or merriment); or any care about or investment in *this* world came, in the first centuries of the Church, to be labeled as manifestations of moral corruption that should be routed out and destroyed. "Mortify the flesh!" soon became the epithet that was believed to capture the core of spiritual wisdom for every devout Christian.

God, the epitome of all that is good, was already described as Pure Reason, Pure Being, indivisible, immutable, invisible, imperturbable, and all powerful.

We, in contrast, in our earthly existence, came to be seen as having life that was besmirched by passion, change, division, fleshly desire, impulse, irrationality, and, worst of all, bodies.

What is ironic about this development is that theologically, the church fathers condemned Docetism (the belief that Christ only *seemed* to have a human body and to suffer and die on the cross) and, later, Gnosticism (the belief that matter is evil) for their radical dualism and elevation of souls over bodies. In so doing, they theoretically affirmed the goodness of creation. Theologically, then, the Fathers got matters right. But in *practice*, the early Church appears to have first condemned Gnosticism and then eaten it, because as it moved resolutely forward, it became increasingly preoccupied with and enamored of souls and increasingly disparaging of bodies and worldliness. This would seem to be a clear proof of Baillie's assertion that "the Church was building better than it knew." Baillie describes this whole development in these words:[2] "The cruder forms of docetism were fairly soon left behind, but in its more subtle forms the danger continued in varying degrees to dog the steps of theology right through the ages until modern times."

As has been said, the seeds of these hellenized philosophical concepts existed in the New Testament itself. Some examples are these: "Do you not know that your body is a temple of the Holy Spirit within you, which you have from God?" (1 Cor. 7); "May the God of peace himself sanctify you wholly; and may your spirit and soul and body be kept sound and blameless" (1 Thess. 5:23); "For this perishable nature must put on the imperishable, and this mortal nature must put on immortality" (1 Cor. 15); " . . . the power of God who abolished death and brought life and immortality to light through the Gospel" (1 Tim. 1:10). Such notions had no comparable influence in the Hebrew Bible, and what is more significant—in fact, crucial—is that they are totally lacking in the sayings of Jesus. This would suggest that the incorporation of these Hellenistic ideas was something that the *Church* did, not a part of what Jesus preached. I will return to this point in a moment, but for now, let us go on and trace where this went in the Christian tradition.

### Hellenization and Asceticism

First, as has been said, as the Christian sect during the first century pulled away from Judaism, it rejected the Jewish view of all things worldly. Cut off from the Jewish zest for life, the body-soul split deepened. Then in 312 A.D. when, almost overnight, Christianity became the official religion of the Roman emperor, its alliance with the Greco-Roman world was sealed. Souls came to be held in higher and higher esteem and bodies viewed as more and more loathsome.

This movement in piety came to be called asceticism and included such practices as total renunciation of worldly possessions, chastity, severe fasting, and sleep deprivation. The movement was given an additional push in the fourth century. In this period, the protracted decline of the Roman Empire and the gross decadence of Roman society led to a general feeling of impending doom. People felt helpless in the face of this cultural and political stagnation that seemed to portend disaster. A retreat to spiritual purity, the urge to flee this world, and a movement toward rigorism were assumed by many to be the only hope. This development dovetailed with the existing body-soul split. (As an aside, it can be noted that the same feeling of malaise plagued Germany in the 1930s. Discontent with society and a generalized yearning for rigorism were seen as the only solution and contributed to the rise of Nazism. In our own day, the same kinds of feelings may be said to have given rise to the radical right.)

### The Trivialization of Immortality

However, while Judaism was held in contempt by the earliest church fathers, there was in Christianity one interweaving of Greek and Jewish thought that produced a strange bolt of cloth. The Greek concept of immortality—which for a Greek, you will remember, was an intangible, distilled apprehension of a sphere of being beyond time—was flattened by Christianity onto the Jewish linear view of life. Immortality for Christians thus mutated into the concept of 'life everlasting' or 'eternal life', which was then understood to mean the time after death tacked onto the end of this time, a continuation of durational time, rather than a dimension of existence beyond time and beyond space. This was, of course, from a Greek point of view, a gross debasement of a highly developed, abstract concept, a rather crass popularization of a highly refined idea. (Incidentally, this development also paved the way for what Father Bede Griffiths has called "surely the most terrible doctrine ever preached by any religion, the doctrine of everlasting punishment."[3])

### The Roots of "The Great By and By"

Another development in the early Church that re-inforced this body-soul split view of the world was the fact that the Second Coming, expected in the life-time of the apostles, did not occur. It is clear from Paul's allusions to it that Jesus' return was expected quite soon and that some of those people who had known Jesus personally, along with new followers of the Way, expected to be "caught up together with [the dead in Christ] to meet the Lord in the air" (1 Thess. 4:17).

When this did not happen, Jesus' promise was pushed into the indefinite future (or in theological talk, eschatologized). Since the future beyond our lifetime was this "life everlasting" or the continued life of the immortal soul, this came to be the longed-for goal. In other words, heaven—the kingdom, the fulfillment of the promise—all got pushed to that time after death.

Consequently, "getting dead" was seen as a won-derful accomplishment. And in fact, martyrdom be-came so popular in the early Church that the first Fathers had to caution the faithful not to seek after it. But this was not intended to blunt death's popularity.

What was to be yearned for above all else was to get this miserable earthly existence over with so that one could dwell in inaccessible light with God.

In terms of how one lived, as long as hopes ran high that Jesus was coming back soon, not investing in worldly things seemed only practical. "Why marry or have children or invest in worldly possessions? Jesus is returning any day now" was the basic stance taken by Paul and most early Christians. But when Jesus did not come, this not investing in worldly things became an ideal and played into the hands of the adopted and modified idea of immortality.

The salient question of the early Church at this point was, How do we live now? Jesus' return was receding into the dim future; the era of martyrdom was over; Judaism had been rejected; Christianity had become the religion of the Greco-Roman empire. What now? What was to be done with the body-soul dichotomy? How was it to be *lived out*?

### Toward the Logical Absurdity

I think it fair to say that martyrdom was replaced in the life of the Church by what came to be called the Counsels of Perfection (basically the religious vows of poverty, chastity, and obedience). The rejection of all bodily things, the demeaning of all earthly things: these developments were part and parcel of Christian theology and piety from the earliest church fathers on. According to Clement of Alexandria (ca. A.D. 200),[4] "to be entirely free from passion is to be most like God Who is impassible." "The perfect man," he says, "is above all affections: courage, fear, cheerfulness, anger, envy, love for the creature." "The saint," says Clement, "is a person who has extirpated his passions." To make pointedly clear how far Christianity had traveled in less than two hundred years, one must realize, of course, that these quotations would have sounded like lunacy to a Jew.

Another example of how this kind of spirituality developed in the Church presents itself in Antony, the desert father and founder of monasticism. By 270 A.D., Antony fully reflected in his life his yearning for a transcendent state and a disdain of the world. His embrace of radical asceticism and renunciation, including severe fasting, abject poverty, self-imposed physical discomforts, celibacy, self-isolation, and the attempt to avoid all earthly pleasures formed the core of his life. They became the cornerstones of monasticism as well.

By the time of Jerome (around 400 A.D.), this tendency to yearn for death and tromp on the body and all sensuous worldly experience had reached its point of logical absurdity. Some choice quotations from Jerome that Kenneth Kirk includes and comments on in *The Vision of God* make this amply clear.[5]

The priest Heliodorus [ordered by Jerome into solitude] . . . is bidden to break away even from [a] slender compromise with the world:

"Should your little nephew hang on your neck, pay no regard to him. Should your mother with ashes on her hair, and garments rent, show you the breasts at which she nursed you, heed her not. Should your father prostrate himself on the threshold, trample him underfoot and go your way. With dry eyes fly to the standard of the cross. In such cases cruelty is the only true kindness. . . . The love of God and the fear of hell will easily break such bonds."

. . . Elsewhere Jerome draws a picture of the "breaking of the bonds"—the departure of the widow Paula from her orphaned children when she set out for the desert:

"The sails were set, and the strokes of the oars carried the vessel into the deep. On the shore the little Toxotius [her son] stretched forth his hands in entreaty; while Rufina, now grown up, with silent sobs besought her mother to wait till she should be married. But still Paula's eyes were dry, as she turned them heavenward. She overcame her love for her children by her love for God."

Apathy towards a death in the family always excited Jerome's warmest approval; where the death was that of a wife or husband he asked for unstinted rejoicing. Blaesilla, Paula's daughter and Eustochium's sister, lost her husband after seven months of married life. "Unhappy girl," Jerome writes, his morbid taste for epigram unblunted even by this tragedy; "You have lost at one and the same time, the crown of virginity and the joys of wedlock." Still, the occasion demands a word of comfort; and he bids her "take heart and rejoice" because she has now "as a widow," the opportunity of exercising "chastity of the lower order." Three months' asceticism under Jerome's guidance brought her to her grave; and Paula her mother suffered a severe rebuke for showing excessive grief; for what Jerome would be prepared to condone in an "average Christian woman" is intolerable in a recluse.

As the brief biography of Jerome included in the Episcopal church's book of *Collects, Psalms and*

*Lessons for the Lesser Feasts and Fasts* concludes, "A militant champion of orthodoxy, an indefatigable worker, and a stylist of rare gifts, Jerome was seldom pleasant, but at least he was never dull."

And what happened to sex and sexuality in the course of all this? Well, of course, they were doomed. Here you have this powerful human appetite leading to sensual pleasure involving the most ardent of bodily human passions. This was the lowest of the low.

Unfortunately, sex could not be eradicated. Chapman Cohen, writing with remarkable astuteness on this topic in 1919, sums it up this way:[6]

The modern history of religion offers a melancholy illustration of the truth of the last sentence [that sex is too potent a reality to ignore], and it is quite clearly exhibited in the history of Christianity itself. From the beginning it strove to suppress the power of sexual feeling. It was an enemy against whom one had to be always on guard, one that had to be crushed, or at least kept in subjection in the interests of spiritual development. And yet the very intensity of the efforts at suppression defeated the object aimed at. With some of the leaders of early Christianity sex became an obsession. Long dwelling upon its power made them unduly and unhealthily conscious of its presence. Instead of sex taking its place as one of the facts of life, which like most other facts might be good or bad as circumstances determined, it was so much dwelt upon as to often dwarf everything else. Asceticism is, after all, mainly a reversed sensualism, or at least confesses the existence of a sensualism that must not be allowed expression lest its manifestation become overpowering. Mortification confesses the supremacy of sense as surely as gratification. Moreover, mortification of sense as preached by the great ascetics does not prevent that most dangerous of all forms of gratification, the sensualism of the imagination.

The uneasy peace that the Church made with what it saw as this despicable sexual appetite rested on its justification for the sake of procreation. From this bizarre point of view, since we clearly had the duty of propagating the race, sex was permissible, but should not be pleasureable. The slightest enjoyment was thought to be sinful. Any form of nonprocreational sex was, of course, anathema.

The Reformation brought some relief from this creation-hating worldview, but not much. The Counsels of Perfection were knocked from their pedestals, it is true. Monasticism (viewed by the Reformers as "works-righteousness" or trying to earn our way into heaven instead of accepting salvation as a gift of God) came to be held in contempt, and married life was retrieved from its status as second best. Luther and his spouse Catherine are known to have much enjoyed connubial bliss; Calvin held a great dance after his wedding. But the hardness of Protestantism simply leaked out in other ways. Because of the Reformation's assumption of the utter depravity of humankind, asceticism continued, only in different forms.

## The Endurance of the Heresy

The point is that this kind of rigorism has waxed and waned in Christianity from Jerome until the present day. There have been Jeromes in every age. De Rancé, for example, the seventeenth-century founder of the Trappists, so ardently wanted his postulants to live holy, disembodied lives that he imposed ascetical rigors on them so severe that they usually died within three years. The puritans reflected the same spirituality in a different social milieu. The Victorians did also, in their own period.

All of these are only extreme manifestations of the same philosophy. The basic tenets remained largely unchallenged, at least until Vatican II. The Christian life at its best came to be characterized as striving toward the soul's release from the prison-house of the body by ascetic practices and self-annihilation. This worldview provided the philosophical underpinnings for the Counsels of Perfection, embodied most fully in religious life as a nun or monk. Such renunciates came to be viewed in the Church as holier than the rest of us because of their more radical rejection of worldly things. After the age of martyrdom had passed, poverty, chastity, and obedience in the monastic setting came to be viewed as *the next best thing to being dead*.

After the Reformation, the radical Anabaptist (envision, if you will, a modern-day Amishman) committed to living a "sober, righteous, and holy life" dramatically exemplified the dedicated Protestant Christian. For those of us who have not been able to manage lives of such rigor, all attempts in the direction of solemnity (manifested as grimness) are judged by the Church as strivings toward holiness.

This, then, has been the orthodox heresy of the Church. A religion was built upon the foundation of a body-soul dualism. Piety came to be defined as a disdain for the world and a yearning for life after death. And these philosophical notions and this ethos are woven into the fabric of our religion and thrive to this very day as we continue to sing,[7]

> Immortal, invisible God only wise,
> Unresting, unhasting and silent as light . . .

Or

> Let all mortal flesh keep silence
> .   .   .   .   .   .   .   .   .   .   .   .   .
> Ponder nothing earthly-minded
> Christ our God to earth descendeth . . .

Or

> Joy that martyrs won their crown
> Opened heav'n's bright portal
> When they laid the mortal down
> For the life immortal.

or whenever we end our prayers, "and bring us to everlasting life." In all of this, we reaffirm our souls as discontinuous from our bodies, our souls as immortal, our bodies as second best, and immortality or heaven as that time of life after death.

Officially, this backdrop still sets the stage for sexual ethics in the teachings of the Roman Catholic church. Marital coitus is declared by Rome to be the only acceptable use of the sexual drive. And in addition, every sexual act must be open to the possibility of procreation, interfered with only by the strange exception of the rhythm method, otherwise known as Vatican roulette, guaranteed to fill with anxiety practically every sexual encounter between husband and wife and thereby dull their pleasure. Masturbation, homosexual intercourse, and nonprocreational forms of heterosexual intercourse are held to be sinful because they have no intrinsic use (read: excuse) except pleasure. And one cannot help but note the marked irrelevance of these philosophical assumptions to the life of the Roman Catholic church in the modern world. The split in the American Catholic church between dogma and practice is a veritable chasm.

Nevertheless, at a subliminal level—and some might own it straight up—I think that many of us still feel we should pay some deference to the Counsels of Perfection: that it is somehow holier (purer) to be nonsexual than sexual; holier (more selfless) to pass up worldly pleasures than to enjoy them; holier (humbler) to deny oneself and submit to someone else—anyone else—than to exercise one's free will. And as for bodies and sex and sensuality, we remain a schizophrenic culture, constantly battling some deep-seated sense of shame about what our bodies are and what they do.

This is where we have been. And so, the heresy is exposed. Correcting it will mean lifting up some other half of the truth. But before proceeding, it would seem that what I have just said should be mitigated somewhat. If I have painted too darkly the historical spirituality of the Church, it is because of the stranglehold it has had on our religion and our lives.

So let me temper my former remarks. I am not saying that the Church's dipping into Greek philosophy per se was bad. Nor am I contending that the body-soul model has been totally without merit in the development of the Church and in the building of the kingdom. But I am saying this: the Church has lifted up a transcendent, otherworldly, disembodied, nonincarnational theology, a theology whose eschatology has been so dominant that for most of us the present is all but completely overshadowed by the future. It has affirmed this half of the truth to the virtual exclusion of its flip side. The Church left behind in the dust the rich Judaic sensuousness that embraces creation as good, and life (mortal life, if you must) as a gift from God. By its preoccupation with the "battle" between our bodies and souls, it has failed to affirm our God-given wholeness. And it has trained us not to see God all around us, but to yearn for Her in some other-worldly abode.

### Reclaiming Our Heritage

The sensuousness of the Hebrew scriptures has always been an embarrassment to the Christian Church.[8] Holy Mother has blushed crimson over the Song of Songs, for instance, which includes such phrases as, "Oh, give me the kisses of your mouth," and "Ah, you are fair, my darling, with your dove-like eyes! Your breasts are like two fawns."[9]

How resolutely has the Church attempted to allegorize away this sensuousness. Bernard of Clairvaux, for example, spent two whole books[10] commenting his way word-by-word through the Song of Songs. His effort was nothing more than a desperate attempt to try to make this book out to be *not* a love song but instead an enormous allegory whose *real* meaning was otherworldly and eschatalogical.

But the Song of Songs *is* a love song, a sensuous, voluptuous, sublime, passionate, embodied, dynamic, gutsy Hebraic torch song. And I wish it could be said that our Jewish forebears included it in the canon of their Scripture precisely because, in this exquisite poetic form, is lifted up the holiness—the sanctity—of sensuousness, the giftedness of embodiment. But it cannot. The Song was a secular poem that was included in the Hebrew Bible only because the rabbis had already allegorized it. So I suppose we will have to be content to thank the Holy Spirit for hoodwinking us all into outsmarting ourselves.

I would contend that this is the half of the truth the Church did *not* lift up, and that in ignoring, or to be more accurate, suppressing this sensuous half of the truth of reality, it has perpetuated a heresy of enormous magnitude for almost two thousand years. Moreover, I believe the Church could be accused of having done a very selective reading of Jesus' words as recorded in Scripture.

As I said earlier, one does not find *anywhere* in Scripture Jesus using Hellenistic language or advocating as the epitome of Christian life asceticism and renunciation of this world. While it is true that Jesus is found going into the desert for long periods and fasting, we also find him repeatedly at feasts, having his head or feet anointed with oil, and associating with people of great wealth. Moreover, not *one* saying of Jesus' includes the words *mortal* or *immortal*. The word *body* occurs only twice, once in Matthew 10 (with a parallel in Luke) where Jesus is quoted to say, "And do not fear those who kill the body but cannot kill the soul; rather fear him who can destroy both soul and body in hell." But if one looks at this saying, Jesus' intent clearly is to mock the dualism to which he alludes (as though he were making reference to a current philosophical fad). He undercuts the soul-body dualism that some unnamed others apparently were affirming. And the only other place where Jesus is said to use the word *body* is in the words of institution, "This is my body," which not only is *not* an affirmation of a body-soul duality, but in fact is the quintessential statement of incarnation and wholeness: in this communing, in my body, all of reality, all of heaven and earth are present.

But what one *does* hear Jesus repeatedly preaching is the inbreaking of this kingdom, this immanent presence of God: " The kingdom of God is at hand" (Matt. 4:17); "The kingdom of God is in the midst of you" (Luke 17:21); "The kingdom of God has come upon you" (Matt. 12:28). Now, these sayings were apparently heard and hence portrayed by the evangelists and Paul as Jesus' talking about *himself*. But as a result of this apparently limited hearing, it can be argued that they missed the *whole* meaning of these sayings. As Reginald Fuller has aptly pointed out, "Jesus pointed to the kingdom and Paul pointed to Jesus."[11]

But that is to say that Paul may only have apprehended *part* of the revelation. While Jesus clearly was *not* saying that He was coterminous with the kingdom (nor would Paul have claimed He was), He indisputably saw Himself as sent by God to usher it in. But what *else* might Jesus have been saying about this kingdom?

It seems to me that Jesus was frequently saying the *reverse* of what the Church *did* in one significant place where it married Judaism and Hellenism. Jesus does not appear to be talking about tacking on eternal life at the end of mortal life. Quite to the contrary, what He appears to be announcing with this kingdom is the infusion of the fullness of life into all spheres of reality. He seems to be saying that *all* of creation is holy; that all that can be apprehended sensuously is sacred; and that God is known potently in all that God creates.

This is a message of radical incarnationalism. Jesus was not telling His friends and relatives to disdain all earthly pleasure and focus on things supernal. Quite the opposite. The *joie de vivre* His co-religionists knew instinctively, Jesus affirmed. But then He went further. In effect He said, "While life in all of its richness is good, I tell you that all of it put together is only the merest hint, only the most passing glimpse, only the most tantalizing foretaste of the consummation of time, of the oneness of space, and of the fullness of joy that transcends time, space, and mortal life and that you shall know after death." In other words, Jesus appears to have been inviting Judaism to stretch itself beyond worldly life as it knew and experienced it—in all of its blessedness—and to see it as an adumbration of the cosmic goodness of God.

## Contemporary Pseudoreforms

We are witnessing in this century a social upheaval of enormous proportions. Behind the unrest are philosophical presuppositions. What is occurring sociologically, I believe, is mostly a rejection of a philosophy that idealizes asceticism. Institutionally, this has manifested itself in the widespread rejection of the Church, which is accurately, if unconsciously, perceived by many to have been the champion of this worldview.

Superficially this may appear to be a liberation from the older ascetic spirit. Morality now seems to be defined no more broadly than "My rights stop where yours start. If my 'thing' doesn't interfere with your 'thing', it's none of your business." Law, in fact, is evolving to embody this philosophy.

Most of America sleeps wherever it wants now, and with whomever it wants. Every possible commodity and personal service, from the ridiculous to the sublime, is available to titillate one's senses. Surely, then, we have thrown off the shackles and become a sensuous society. Surely *now* we have reclaimed the sensuousness portrayed in the Hebrew scriptures.

Oh yes, it is true that earlier, in the sixties and somewhat in the seventies, this liberation movement began as a rather petulant, adolescent rebellion. But now, in the eighties, it is all grown up. This is the decade of the upwardly mobile, of the fit, of the strivers for excellence. Surely we are now worthy of being called liberated.

If we were a more peaceful nation, a more loving society, a more caring people, our presumed claim to wholeness would be more convincing, at least to me. But the fact is, the "liberation" achieved in the past thirty years has been no more integrative than the ascetic approach it rejected.

Nor have the basic philosophical underpinnings

been overthrown. The body-soul dualism is still firmly in place. The body and sensuousness are still exclusively associated with the ungodly (secular) world; the soul with the religious (sacred). The only difference is that now the scales have been tipped. Now bodies and sensuousness and secularism reign supreme, while religion and spiritual things mostly are held in ridicule as quaint archaisms, consigned, along with other activities of "primitive man," to the cultural anthropology departments of most universities.

What we see, then, in the Western world today is a kind of sensualism gone wild. It is a reactionary philosophy that would replace asceticism with hedonism. If the eighties are all grown up, they are just as self-indulgent as the seventies and sixties were, and, in fact, just as self-preoccupied as eras that committed themselves to the ascetical way.

In response to this hedonistic reactionism, a conservative minority (the Counter-Reformation of the eighties) is determined to reinstate the former status quo. They condemn, in a way that would warm any Puritan's heart, all sensuous pleasure. These Bible-thumping, literalist rigorists are doling out in modern garb, under the banner of "family-centeredness" and "wholesomeness," nothing more than antisepticized reality, life disembodied from any real passion or sensuousness. The radical right, then, offers just more of the same tired old asceticism in a new habit. And at the same time, in the Roman camp, we have seen, of late, an appalling resurgence of Vatican autocracy, including insistence upon some very tired and irrelevant dogmas coupled with some incredibly heavy-handed discipline visited upon those sons of Rome who do not wholeheartedly assent.

And in the middle are the rest of us confused Christians, wondering what to do and knowing that both the hedonistic reactionaries and the counterreformers are wrong. In the pits of our stomachs, we know that in their fanaticism they are both perpetuating heresy.

What still has not been tried is a *sacralization* of sensuousness. This would require coming to know all of creation as holy. And this attitude is not much in evidence in the United States of the 1980s, certainly not among the Radical Sensualists or the Radical Rightists.

### Some Rays of Hope

However, within mainline Christianity during the past thirty years, we have seen the proliferation of new and exciting theologies that seem to offer great promise. What do they reflect of the spiritual life of the Church? It would seem that these new theologies are serving to dethrone the rigorist, fragmenting, lopsided, quasi-Greek philosophical ideals from their long-unchallenged reign as the sole foundations of Christian theology by offering something *positive* with which to supplement them.

Process theology has knocked the slats out from under the portrait of the immutable, indivisible, unmoved-mover God of Whom we have been so fond, and has declared God to be all-dynamic and manifest in diversity as well as unity. Liberation theology has insisted that we see God infused into *this* life, this wholly mortal life; that we see wordly life as a locus where God is integrally involved and passionately interested. In the spiritual sphere, Matthew Fox and his "creation-centered" troop may border on being what I characterize as "bliss-ninnies," but they do breathe some much-needed fresh air of joyful embodiment into the Church as an antidote to the former grim world of ascetic spirituality. And finally, theologians like James Nelson[12] and feminist theologians and gay theologians are forcing the Church to deal with our bodies as part of our wholeness, and our corporeality as sacred.

I see the current libertarianism of our society and the radical theologizing within the Church as comprising a blessed heresy that, I will admit, is being asserted with all of the hair-raising vengeance of the sixteenth-century Reformers, but that is a Godsend nonetheless. It appears to have been sent to the Church to cleanse it, to correct a deeply ingrained error that has been perpetuated for many centuries and that has caused much spiritual damage.

I believe we face more unsettled times ahead as this spiritual continental shift works its way to the surface. Most reforms go too far, which then require a time of balancing, of coming to a settlement (something my own Anglican church has a long history of being good at). And then the possibility of re-evangelization will present itself, as we, a chastened church, call the world to a new and more complete spiritual vision. It will not be easy. We have offered so little for so long.

But ultimately I believe we will end up a healthier Church if we succeed. We will be a people that lifts up the *whole* truth about life immanent and life transcendent, so that eventually we will be able to raise up, without a hint of embarrassment, the words of the Song of Songs

> I have come to my garden,
> My own, my bride;
> I have plucked my myrrh and spice,
> Eaten my honey and honeycomb,
> Drunk my wine and my milk.
>
> Eat, lovers, and drink:
> Drink deep of love!

and not experience these evocative expressions as some sort of soft pornography, but affirm them with all our hearts as a sublime and sacred articulation of sensuous love, which is, I am sure, how God hears them.

# CHAPTER 3

# The Dilemma

Against the confusing spiritual backdrop of the United States in the 1980s described in chapter 2, with all of its conflictedness about sensuality, pleasure, bodies, death, and sex, AIDS made its entrance.

## *A Tray of Shattered Fantasies*

Most everyone would agree that it could not have come at a worse time. Here we had almost succeeded in obliterating death from our consciousnesses. We had worked so hard and for so long. More than a century of progressively hiding the Grim Reaper, of euphemizing death, of phoneying up corpses, of putting fake grass around the hole and leaving before the box was lowered. We had almost secreted ourselves from death, almost antisepticized it. And we were within a hair's breadth of our goal.

A culture of vigor and zest and health is what we fancied ourselves. Fitness and preventive medicine, organic food and vitamins and macrobiotics, Nautilus and Jazzercise, *Prevention* magazine and *Runner's World*. Eighty year olds winning marathons. And compared with just ten years ago, 60 percent more senior citizens with natural teeth instead of dentures.

If Ponce de Leon's fountain of youth had not quite

been found, if Dr. Faust's formula for everlasting human life had not actually been discovered, we could deceive ourselves across the insignificant gap that remained. Oh, such a tiny little gap it was between old-age vigor (which we were sure we could have—*every single one of us*) and embodied immortality.

And then some of our brothers, many in the glowing vigor of youth, including many an iron pumper, many a health food eater, and many a tooth flosser, started wasting away.

It could not have come at a worse time. Western medicine seemed to be reaching its zenith. The hard sciences, technology, and human inventiveness were proving to be our *real* messiahs: artificial hearts and bionic limbs, wonder drugs and CAT scans, childhood diseases all but licked, a cure for multiple sclerosis so close we could taste it, cancer on the run, spliced genes promising yet more medical miracles, and life spans edging upward nicely.

And then a fragile little bug snuck its way into some of our bloodstreams and began its deadly dance. Neither any hard science nor technology nor human inventiveness had the hint of an *answer*, let alone a promise of salvation. Hell, for the first year or so, no one could even formulate the right *question*. Our Science God caught short, embarrassed, exposed in all of its too-smallness.

It could not have come at a worse time. Hard-won gay rights had been gained. We had almost bullied our way into the club. We were doctors, lawyers, priests, and politicians now. Protective laws were springing up like weeds. The love that once had dared not speak its name had become the love that would not shut up: hundreds of books and movies and documentaries and conventions and clubs and choruses and soaps and even representation on "Dynasty." Gay gentrification and upward mobility. A guppie for every yuppie. Equal opportunity to pursue the great American bitch-goddess almost in our grip.

And then they said it was contagious. And that we gay men had a great deal of it. And now employers, the Joint Chiefs of Staff, the Supreme Court, and insurance companies yearn for the good old days. There's talk of quarantines and mandatory screening. And now a big rock alongside the Pennsylvania Tunpike has painted on it, "KILL AIDS, KILL GAYS" and some fine upstanding American citizens are doing it.[1]

Here we had almost succeeded in reducing religion to an aesthetic experience, a mélange of opera, museum, and botanical garden, a thing to be pursued *chacun à son goût*, an unnecessary but refined undertaking, or conversely, a way to get weekly warm fuzzies.

The pursuit of justice needed no help from a god; the courts could manage. Ethics could survive without a deity as well. The media had monopolized ritual. Charity in any embodied form had passed largely into the institutional hands of the welfare system. Science had explained away what might have been miraculous and would demythologize the rest soon enough. And who needed religion to explain death when we had stopped acknowledging that human beings have a 100 percent mortality rate?

Edward Shils in his book *Tradition*[2] had this to say

about death's denial and Christianity's demise:

Death, at least on the conscious level, is not as salient nowadays in Western societies as it was several centuries ago. It has become . . . a less continuously obtruding problem. . . . The great improvements in preventive medicine and in surgery and the increased consumption of nutritive foods have fortified the hope of remaining alive, or postponing death so that the thought of it can be put aside. The problems which the Christian conceptions of death and immortality treated, being terrifyingly painful problems and difficult to face, have been illusorily averted and put out of mind by many persons in contemporary Western societies. As a result, the Christian traditions regarding mortality and immortality have been attenuated. . . . The traditional Christian interpretation of death was of course a grander and graver tradition than the traditions of socialism and liberalism [that replaced it]. The fact of death is, in a certain sense, a deeper fact than the fact of material well-being. Nonetheless, it has been relegated, very uneasily and unsatisfyingly, to a less prominent position. It has therefore changed the pattern of the Christian tradition for many of its adherents.

. . . at least until AIDS. And now, with a vengeance whose magnitude is in inverse and equal proportion to the willfulness with which we played God and thumbed our noses at mortality, it confronts us. We were not prepared for this. And if "how it feels" is used as a basis for judging, one must say "it could not have come at a worse time."

### In Search of The Meaning of AIDS

But perhaps, just perhaps, "how it feels" is *not* the right criterion for judging. And maybe making the problem go away is not the profoundest answer. And if not, then what is?

Everything means something: that is the therapist in me speaking. And the resident theologian cannot help but try to see everything somehow as part of God's unfolding of Her universe. If not, God is not God, contemporary Western society has been right, and we believers truly *are* fools.

So what does AIDS mean? What does it mean for our spiritual journeys—those of us who have it and those of us who do not; those of us who are gay and those of us who are not? What does it mean? How does it fit? How do we make sense of society's violent reaction to this disease? To people with AIDS? To gay people since AIDS appeared? What is God up to? Can we even know?

The only clues I have been able to find in my attempts to read these entrails, in trying to decipher these runes, have come from my own journey of this past year, a slice of my life that, until now, has been too close to home and too fresh to tell. Like effective poetry, stories—especially personal ones—have got to be matters of "emotion recollected in tranquility" or they help no one. I think my story is clean now, and it feels too important in this context *not* to share. But I will have to be careful nonetheless, because I will be working from analogy, and analogies are always faulty . . . and dangerous.

What it means actually to *have* AIDS, I cannot know, any more than I can know what it means to be a woman, or black, or heterosexual. No matter how much I try, by analogy with things in my life, to get what it would be like to have AIDS, I will never achieve more than an approximation. So if I am way off, my brothers and sisters with AIDS, I apologize.

### Personal Saga: A Journey into Illness

This past year, God gave me a gift, although it has taken a year to know it as a gift. In March 1985, I got ill. Not very ill, not gravely ill, but ill enough to be almost dysfunctional. Flu-like symptoms: malaise, fevers, listlessness, incredible achiness, clamminess, sweatiness, sore throats, and other weird things.

The symptoms lasted. And lasted. Weeks turned into months. Physician succeeded physician—eight in all. My blood was mostly all right: slightly elevated white cell count. But I looked healthy. And I was gaining weight.

Diagnoses went from "a virus" in April, to "stress" in June, to "psychosomatic illness or hypochondria" in August. This was an unfortunate sequence, enough almost to jade me on American medicine. I knew *me* pretty well, body and soul. I knew this was not stress. And I knew I was no hypochondriac. Crazy, yes; hypochondriacal, no. It felt increasingly, as medical attempts at discovery repeatedly failed, that I was being blamed for having the effrontery to contract a disease for which no one could find a name. It seemed to offend people's self-esteem, which in itself is a sad commentary on how physicians have bought into playing the god people want them to be.

Under all my other feelings was the terror that I had *it*, the Big A. Or if not AIDS itself, something just as terrifying. Even though my blood did not prove it (yet), what my head kept telling me was, "I've got this illness that won't go away. My body's not fighting it off," which seemed to be the same as, "My immune system isn't working. Why? O God, why?" A continuous-loop tape that played and played, constantly, either in the foreground or background of my life.

March to October without a name for it. Seven months of obsessing, of psychic immobilization, of nightmares, of visiting friends from far away and thinking, "God, it's good to see them 'one more time.'" Months of feeling unable to invest in what seemed—however imagined—like a very short future.

Eventually in my grieving travels, I reached the stage that Elisabeth Kübler-Ross calls bargaining. I dug in my heels. I stopped publicly speaking, wrote nary a word, and for a while, stayed home Sunday mornings. I'd show Him. I even passed up a 90-percent scholarship to the University of Chicago Divinity School. In effect, I shook my fist at God, clenched my teeth, set my jaw, and seethed, "Until you give me my health back, you can take your kingdom and stuff it!"

It wasn't fair, you see. I ate right. I slept enough. I took vitamins. I had had seven years of psychotherapy, and even stress management training. I ran three to five miles a day. I was a professional in the prime of life. And I had spent ten years out there on the bleeding edge of reality, trying to help God move this reticent Church toward the Parousia. And so I dug in my heels. And I *sat*, righteous and wounded.

In November, a Chicago legend named Jakub Schlichter—a seventy-four-year-old Viennese internist with a Yiddish accent you could cut with a machete—

agreed to see me. I had never had a three-hour examination or seen anyone wield a fine-toothed comb with quite such panache.

The second appointment went something like this. "Good news and bad news," began Schlichter. (You'll have to imagine the accent.) "First, your AIDS antibodies test was negative and your T-cells look terrific. I'd give you 99 percent you've never met the virus. So stop worrying about *that* already. On the other hand, your titers for Epstein-Barr virus is quite high. And your mono spot is negative. Having ruled everything else out, and with the symptoms you've got and for as long as you've had them, some people are saying this is a chronic form of mono. But nobody knows for sure," he said. "And even if it is, there's no cure and not much treatment." Then he leaned forward, looked me right in the eye, and pronounced with unmitigated finality, "You're going to have to learn to live with this."

"You're going to have to learn to live with this." Words that fell like a sheet of lead on my back. I went numb.

The rage did not arrive until several hours later. Live with it! This was insult to injury. Having endured the agony of not knowing for seven months, now all I knew was that I was probably going to feel rotten for the rest of my life. Like hell.

And so I sat some more. Righteous and wounded and now *mad*. And, in case She had missed it, I told that Divine Vivisector one more time, "Until you give me my health back, I quit. You got it? You're on your own!"

And out of the prolonged silence that ensued (a silence of months—I am *very* stubborn) . . . came an answer. A still small voice, maybe. (It is strange how God, like Schlichter, always talks to me with a Yiddish accent.) And He said just this: "So how long can you hold your breath, already?"

What's a guy to do? I decided we'd do it God's way—this time. And so I gave up. And I got up. And I got on with my life: counseling and speaking and writing—and oh, by the way, the University of Chicago had saved my scholarship for me. Chance? I think not.

But life is different now. And that is mostly the point of my story, although from tales they tell me, the process that people with AIDS go through on the way toward getting on with their lives seems very similar to mine. But life is qualitatively different now, and that is the main point. I would be a liar if I said I am no longer stubborn. But I feel older now, and wizened, and in some strange way, more peaceful.

Feeling chronically like you have the flu (and that is how it is for me nowadays) is not the same as having a disease that most often kills within two years. I don't know what it's like to face that—I only *tasted* that. But I can tell you that chronic illness does make one very aware of one's mortality. All the time. I can no longer live as though this life were forever; I can no longer, as Shils captured it, "put death aside," because I am, moment by moment, reminded by my body that it is on the way. And from things they tell me, my brothers and sisters with AIDS apparently know this feeling, too.

This illness has had a second major effect on my life as well. I used to live so much in the future. Hopes and dreams, fears and schemes. Like Annie taught us, "Tomorrow, tomorrow, I love ya, tomorrow . . ."

No more. I no longer have the energy for it. Knowing that there is an *end* changes everything. It makes this moment—this moment, when I happen to be sitting here writing—but this moment, whatever moment it may be—so very important. I want it in its fullness; I want all it holds. It is not so much that I want to slow things down as that I want not to miss any moment's essence. And my brothers and sisters with AIDS seem to know *this* feeling acutely.

One of them, a historian friend named Jack Balcer, having taken what might well be his last trip to Italy, wrote this to me when he returned:

Spring is here, and I have had the good fortune of seeing it, feeling it, being in it, sitting in it, as it began in Tuscany and Florence . . . there I was. My trip was fantastic. Now, I garden to my delight and continue my Greek-Persian studies. It is still April and it feels like June. What will July and August bring? Be well, enjoy, drop me a card now and then. Buona Primavera.

Of course, this living profoundly in the moment is no *new* piece of wisdom. It is only new for me. The eminent theologian Karl Rahner wrote this about the topic:[3]

If we look at this life of ours, it is of itself *not* of such a nature that one would like to go on forever here; of itself, it strives toward a conclusion to its present mode of existence. *Time becomes madness* if it cannot reach fulfillment. To be able to go on forever would be the hell of empty meaninglessness. No moment would have any importance because one could postpone and put everything off until an empty later which would always be there.

Time becomes madness. The hell of empty meaninglessness. No moment having any importance. Postponing everything until an empty later. Do these phrases strike any chords in you, surrounded as we are by cocaine-induced stupors and brain-wave-jamming megadecibel music, life in the fast lane, one's soul harnessed to a computer monitor, teenage suicides, and young upwardly mobiles too emotionally deadened by the cost of ambition to enjoy sex, let alone the Porsche?

Living as though death were a myth robs life of its conclusion. And the madness is all about us. Or so it seems to me.

### Proclaiming The Good News of Mortality

While it may not be fair, it always seems to be those who are oppressed who must lead the Church and society toward whatever revelation they must embrace next. I had always seen our prophetic role as gay men and lesbians to be leading the Church and Western civilization toward re-embracing our embodiedness, toward a recovery, if you will, of Holy Sensuousness, which, as we saw in chapter 2, has been systematically suppressed by a Church much taken with a Hellenized body-soul duality and then perpetuated by Western civilization in one form or another.

I still think that lifting up the sacredness of creation is part of our call. As we have seen, it is still a piece of reality that Church and society largely ignore. And it would certainly seem that one of the reasons the Church and Western society are so threatened by gay people is that in our sexuality there is not the excuse of procreation that the Church has often used grudgingly to permit the pleasure of sex: "Better to marry than to burn." Our sexuality is patently worldly, which may be why we have so often been labeled flighty, immature, self-indulgent, hedonistic—all terms a creation-hating, otherworldly imprisoned society might use to express its envy.

But what I had *not* seen before my illness is that to affirm sensuousness is to run headlong into death. To live fully in one's body is to experience that sooner or later this body will rot. Whether it is taut and muscled or fat and flabby, it will rot. *None of us is getting out of this alive.* If one opts *not* to live life as though one were almost already a disembodied spirit, then the alternative, living embodied—sensuously—means that you must always deal with death lurking in the shadow.

There is a sense in which gay people have always represented mortality to the world: deeply, darkly, archetypally. Since in our sexuality we are patently nonprocreational, we intimate death to people. We are after all—most of us—the ends of our family trees. Not to make babies is to make not-babies. And not-birth is experienced at some primordial level as death.

We are not alone in this. Nonprocreating people have often frightened the world, especially in scary times. If a nonbearing wife of ancient Israel, when survival of the clan seemed tenuous, then one was seen as cursed; if one of a group of sixteenth-century religious under vows when the medieval world was falling apart, then suppressed; if an old spinster in the turbulent times of Puritan England or New England, labeled a witch; and if gay or lesbian in these disintegrative days of the twentieth century, then diagnosed as a pervert, invert, character disorder, borderline personality, or condemned as a Sodomite or abomination against God. There are such a wondrous variety of us.

And now we who are gay, who at some subliminal level already intimate death to people, now we have been linked in the public's mind with a frightening, mostly fatal disease. It is a deadly combination. It has made us expedient scapegoats, because we and AIDS, and especially the synergistic combination, remind a society bulwarked against death of their inevitable ends. How rude.

Perhaps this is the fullness of the revelation that the Divine Nudge intends for us who are gay and lesbian to proclaim to the world: the truth of Holy Mortality. In light of the madness that death's denial is wreaking on the world, it would seem to be a truth the world needs to hear.

Gay people have long proclaimed at least half the truth of mortality—the half that gives us such voracious appetites for life. It is an appetite that many oppressed people seem to develop, maybe because life on the fringes always feels so tenuous.

I remember back in the early seventies, a black feminist friend of mine named Geraldine and I were comparing notes on gay and black liberation. "Honey," she said, "there's one basic thing you-all and we-all have in common." "What's that, Geraldine?" I asked. "Darlin'," she said, "we both teach them honkies how to boogey." And she was right. We *do* relish the good life.

The writer of Ecclesiastes couched mortality in about the same terms. "Go, eat your bread with joy," he wrote, "and drink your wine lustily. Let your clothes be fresh and clean and your head oiled." (I suppose today, he would have written *moussed*.) "Enjoy happiness with someone you love," he wrote, "all the fleeting days of life that have been granted you under the sun, before the day comes when your dust returns to the earth it came from, and your breath to God who gave it to you, while your mourners are already back walking to and fro in the streets."

There is elegance and truth in this worldview: there is sanity in living this limited life as fully as one can. This is a truth I have glimpsed now, thanks to the Epstein-Barr syndrome with which I live. It is a truth many of my brothers and sisters with AIDS seem to understand, too. I have never known a more spiritually present bunch. And I believe that when Jesus talked about wanting us to have life abundantly, and about the kingdom of God being in the midst of us, he meant for us very much to cherish this time, this space, this creation, in all of its glorious sensuousness.

As we have seen, the Church has not been much inclined to hear Jesus' words in this way during its first two thousand years. In its eschatological zeal, it has often been disdainful of the world. And in this, as

I said earlier, it has been very wrong. Perhaps in *our* penchant for play, in our zest for life, we who "know how to boogey" shall tease this crusty old Church into embracing the happy, joyful truth about the sanctity of sensuousness.

But we who are gay also, I think have been blind to that *other* part of the truth. For if we stop with *this* life, this half of the truth, if we live as though life were no more than we see and death the bitter end, then gay people do indeed point to a terrible reality, which may explain in part the cynicism or jadedness (what gets referred to in the gay community as being a "bitchy old queen") that has not been uncommon among senior gays.

Without the hope that comes from Jesus' promise that there is *more* than what we see or know, the best we will ever manage in our human existence is courageous despair, a world of "eating, drinking, and being merry, because . . . " Well, you know the rest.

There must be *more* than boogeying, because there is an *end* to boogeying, and then what? There must be more than drinking wine lustily, because wineskins inevitably run dry. The writer of Ecclesiastes, who held no eschatological hope, ultimately succumbs to such despair. His final words, after all, are "Vanity of vanities. All is vanity!" which is better rendered into modern English as, "Futility of futilities. All is futility!"

We Christians claim that death is not the end, that it is only a dark portal leading to the fullness of life. A mysterious reality, of which we catch only glimpses. And if truth be told, most of us spend our lives waffling somewhere between doubt and faith.

But eternal joy is what Jesus came to tell us about. The kingdom is what He preached. Paradise is what He promised.

As I said in chapter 2, in all of His kingdom talk, while Jesus clearly was not telling His fellow Jews to disdain this world, He *was* pointing beyond it. He began where they were: "Yes," He said in effect, "life is good. Drink it to its dregs. It is a gift to you. Enjoy the pleasures that your senses make possible: good food and wine and music and making love with the one you love. Live each moment in all of its pregnancy."

All this Jesus' fellow Jews already knew. They still do. Schlichter knows it. "So I'm not dying," I said to him. "Death?" Schlichter said disdainfully. "The hell with death. You only have two choices: living or not living. Take your pick."

But then, as we have seen, Jesus said more, more than most of His Jewish brothers and sisters could fathom. He preached that there are no limits to this reality—that it transcends time, it transcends space, it transcends birth and death—but that it is completely infused in them as well.

This is the vision to which Jesus beckoned His fellow Jews. He invites us to share it, too. *This* is the other half of the truth that mortality illuminates. And Shils was right about it. Compared with this grand and grave Christian understanding of life and death, the material well-being promised by socialism or liberalism (by radical rightism or upward mobility) looks sordid, paltry, and trite. And only a culture as egoma-

niacal as ours could have tossed the former aside so
cavalierly.

### Grace Amid The Anguish

I posed a question earlier: What is the meaning of
AIDS? It is a cosmic kind of question, bordering on the
rhetorical. Rationally, I cannot comprehend the why
of AIDS. I do not know why ten thousand of my brothers and sisters have had to die of it, fifteen of whom I
have called friend. I do not know why people who
regularly need blood, hence already suffering from
some frightening disease, have had to have insult added to injury. I cannot fathom why innocent children
and infants have had to die painful deaths at AIDS's
hands. And closer to my home, I do not know why
God—whose ways I wish I could just give up trying
to understand—initially chose gay men to comprise
most of AIDS's victims. Some days it seems so awfully
cruel. Merciful God, have we not suffered enough?

So lacking a reasonable answer, I will make a stab
at a *nonrational* answer to the why of AIDS. And it is
this. If our journey with AIDS serves to bring us all
home to the grand and grave, the joyful and sobering
truth of our mortality; if this suffering helps heal the
madness of an eternally empty later whose existence
we have duped ourselves into believing in; if this
nightmare brings back to our consciousness the resurrection hope without which life is just so much courageous despair, then in this groaning of creation,
with tears and sighs, perhaps the Holy Spirit will

usher in some modicum of peace or even a corner of salvation that might otherwise have been unattainable. And in that travail, perhaps . . . perhaps we will glimpse the meaning of AIDS for our spiritual journeys.

I see signs of such a coming dawn. I see some of America's best instincts being evoked in this sad ordeal. The Rabid Right's declaration that AIDS is God's judgment on gay people for their sinfulness has served to toll its own death knell. This grotesque perversion of Jesus' message of compassion that markets itself under the guise of born-again Christianity has now shown itself for what it is; its paper-thin pseudo-Christian mask has slipped. Its day is passing as we watch. I am sure of it. In fact, in response to this outrageous allegation, an Episcopal bishop quipped recently that "if AIDS is indeed retribution from God against gay people, then shouldn't the perpetrators of terror, war, torture, and oppression in the world at least get herpes?"

America's compassion is being evoked in this crisis as well. Its sense of fair play and its hatred of mean-heartedness simply will not tolerate a man being kicked when he is down.

In an incredibly poignant story in the *Chicago Tribune*[4] recently, a heterosexual medical student named Ben Kemena explored the gut-wrenching conflicts he experienced when he was assigned a young gay AIDS patient during his internship. He owns in this article his unwillingness during that period, while on rounds, to say much about his patient to his colleagues "lest [his] remarks be misinterpreted as enthusiasm for this homosexual patient." But he also confesses now, "James was gay, and something about that still prejudiced me. But he was sharp, witty and optimistic, and I admired that. I caught myself wondering how I could admire someone who was homosexual."

Kemena goes on to tell about his relief when James was temporarily discharged from the hospital, first because he would no longer be confronted with his own homophobia, but also because he was "getting tired of being heckled by [his] classmates and residents as the unfortunate medical student who 'got stuck with an AIDS patient.' "

James of course was readmitted to the ward, in terrible agony, as he approached death:

I reached over and touched his arm, and he looked at my hand. "I know I must look horrible since you last saw me," James mumbled. "But don't worry, the morphine is working and I feel a lot better than when I came in last night. The pain has been awful. Someone said my intestines got blocked."

I felt tears forming and wiped my eyes quickly. I had never cried in front of a patient, and I did not want to start. I felt so many emotions. No human deserved this . . . I cared about James, and right then, I felt a love for him.

There is a new and palpable softening of the attitude of American society toward gay people. I swear it is in the air. In light of it, last year's Supreme Court decision upholding Georgia's sodomy statute and the Vatican's attempts to reassert its former moribund stance on sexual ethics seem only like the last throes of a dying paradigm.

But there is other evidence as well. The Episcopal

church in the fall of 1985 came to within a handful of votes of affirming the worthiness of openly gay people for ordination. Just six years earlier, it had overwhelmingly opposed it. This is a chastened Church; these are opening hearts. In fact, these are all hopeful signs. But will our liberation have to be bought at so dear a price, good Lord?

And in the gay community itself, there is grace amid all this pain. We are learning that liberation means more than license. It is dawning on us that loving is not the same as falling in love, let alone making love; and that the price of loving is high, though its dividends are great. But did it have to take this wretched virus to lead us into deeper intimacy with each other and you, merciful God?

I began these remarks with the words, "It could not have come at a worse time." That was a foil, of course, a rhetorical tool to expose some of society's ills. Yet, I cannot in the end bring myself to say its opposite, to say, "It could not have come at a *better* time," no matter how much grace flows through this time of trial. I could not wish any of the pain of AIDS on anyone. And I pray for nothing more fervently than a cure and vaccine, and an end to this nightmare.

But in the end, my faith demands that I say this much: this is all in God's hands. And so, in some incomprehensible way, it must have to be as it is. And if there is no ready answer, no logical explanation for the pain of those dying, for the fear of those who are ill, for the grief of those left behind—if there is no *answer*, there is for us assuredly a *response*.

We must love each other through this, for if

compassion is not the most human of responses, then there is no hope. We must love each other through this, because all we have is each other. We must love each other through this—bearing one another's pain, and affirming for each other the promise that neither death nor life; nor angels, nor principalities; neither things present, nor things to come; neither Kaposi's nor pneumocystis, nor any syndrome nor anguish nor pain, nor the hatred of those who fear us; nor anything else in all creation, can separate us from the love of God or keep us from the kingdom prepared for us from the beginning of the world.

How can this bearing of pain and this affirming of the promise be made manifest among us? How do we move these phrases from being consoling words to tangible realities? The remainder of this book will address those challenges.

# CHAPTER 4

## Bearing the Pain

A colleague once suggested a distinction that I have always found useful between the words *pain* and *suffering*.[1] He noted that pain—the pure experience of it—is open, airy, dynamic, energizing, cleansing, and bright. Suffering he defined as our resistance to pain, our bracing ourselves against it. And in this refusal to let the pain *be*, suffering takes on a closed, fetid, debilitating quality. I find this a helpful way to look at things.

### A Conundrum: When to Surrender

Pain is a fact of life. Some of us may be presented with more of it than others, although this would be hard to substantiate. Does my pain hurt me worse than yours hurts you? Is your physical pain more painful than my mental anguish? How could we quantify these experiences in order to compare them?

The inclination to quantify levels of pain is already a movement toward suffering. In order to quantify something (to think about how much of it there is), we must fix it in our minds. This interruption of its flow continues while we compare it to other pains ("I've never endured such agony before"; "Nobody has ever had to go through the likes of *this*"). Can't you already feel the pall settling over the scene? The life in the pain has stagnated, the windows have been shuttered. The only thing left to do is to sit and wallow in it.

And yet, suffering seems to be a reflexive human response. At the first hint of pain—in fact, at the first anticipation of it—we automatically seem to assume one of two primordial stances, flight or fight. We seem compelled either to try to escape the pain or to pit ourselves against it.

These knee-jerk reactions to painful situations would seem to arise out of our old brains, evolutionarily the most primitive parts of our encephela from which instinctive behaviors barrel forth. We see the same behaviors in our more primitive mammalian relatives. Your cats or dogs will demonstrate them for you with very little provocation.

Your dogs or cats, however, will also demonstrate for you another primitive kind of behavior when it becomes apparent to them that neither fight nor flight is possible. Especially in the face of severe physical pain and, in particular, imminent death, animals tend simply to lie down and *be*. They are clearly in pain: they wheeze or sigh or emit other sounds of pain. But they generally do not shriek; they mostly seek quiet, secluded places; and then they simply live the inescapable experience of pain and dying. They do not seem resentful about it; they do not seem to resist it. They seem just to do what the moment requires.

The difficulty for humankind is that, in addition to our possession of these old, instinctive responses, we also are sentient, self-conscious beings. We have, relatively speaking, enormous cognitive power resident in our new brains, our cerebral cortices. We not only experience pain, something all living creatures with nervous systems appear to do; we also reflect on our experience of pain. We remember pains of the past; we ponder former agonies; we replay miseries we have watched others undergo.

We develop, then, a stance toward any anticipated pain. So when a new pain comes along, our ever-active new brains cannot allow us simply to *be* in this pain. Our set toward pain, coupled with our reliance on cognitive human technological wonders like modern medicine and our remarkable ability to engage in abstract thought of an imaginative and religious nature all conspire to allow us to *extend* the old-brain commitment to fight or flee. In other words, unlike any other earthly creature, we can delay surrendering to the pain virtually to the moment of death, if it comes to that: we can go down fighting. This is a uniquely human behavior.

In a way, it is futile to criticize ourselves for being this way. After all, we are not *not* human. And it is not bad to enjoy well-being and life and to want to maximize both. This is an altogether creaturely desire, or else the flight and fight responses would not be so universal in the animal world. But our determination not to let pain *be* puts us in a fix: it consigns us to a great deal of suffering.

Our dilemma has to do with the degree of stubbornness with which we try to escape or engage in battle in the face of life's distresses. And AIDS, because it is a painful phenomenon from almost any

angle, has made obvious the depth of our commitment to avoiding pain as well as the almost certain
suffering we build into our dealing with the inescapable loss of life to which AIDS leads.

How might we deal better with this pain? How
might we curtail the suffering? How could we use at
least some of the excruciation of AIDS to produce
spiritual growth?

### Wrestling with Paradoxes

It is my perception that if we wish to reach spiritual equanimity with AIDS, we must each wrestle with
the pain of it to the point of surrender. And this is to
tangle in one's guts with a fundamental paradox.

In the East, sparring with a paradox to achieve
spiritual growth is precisely what sayings called koans
are intended to provoke. A koan is a frequently para-
doxical saying given by a Zen master to disciples to
train them to abandon ultimate dependence on reason, thereby forcing them into gaining sudden intuitive enlightenment. An ancient Zen master describes
a koan in these words:

The *koan* is a torch of wisdom that lights up the darkness
of feeling and discrimination, a golden scraper that cuts
away the film clouding the eye, a sharp ax that severs the
root of birth and death, a divine mirror that reflects the
original face of both the sacred and the secular.[2]

Some examples of koans are these:[3]

When an ordinary man attains knowledge he is a sage;
when a sage attains understanding he is an ordinary man.

Who is the teacher of all the Buddhas, past, present, and future? John the cook.

Lo, a cloud of dust is rising from the ocean, and the roaring of the waves is heard over the land.

When both hands are clapped a sound is produced: listen to the sound of one hand.

On the surface, these statements seem like enigmatic, sometimes illogical gibberish. The rational mind wants to dismiss them and move on. But a Zen master will carefully choose a koan for a student and require him or her to sit and comtemplate on the unnerving collection of words. The student will undoubtedly try harder and harder to make sense of the koan . . . and will fail. And at the moment of failing—of giving up—he or she will (hundreds of years of Zen practice affirm) spontaneously achieve some piece of spiritual enlightenment. This enlightenment may superficially seem unrelated to the actual words of the koan. No matter. If it has led the student deeper, it will have been useful. One thing, however, is always true of the contemplation of koans: the enlightenment reached could never have been logically adduced from the words given.

In Christian symbolism, the cross has long been an object of Christian contemplation, especially at certain times of the year. It is the symbol of the Crucifixion in all of its ugliness, all of its agony, all of its absurdity. It seems to me that the Crucifixion is the ultimate Christian paradox, the paramount Christian koan. And the purpose of contemplating the paradox of the cross is and has always been to achieve spiritual growth.

No matter who you are or what you believe, the cross makes no sense. Whether you look at it as a non-believing student of religion and see the primordial earth-father demanding the sadistic execution of his own son as compensation for the mess he himself made in concocting humanity; or as a humanist and see simply a good and zealous man allowing himself, for a cause, to be brutally murdered when he could have avoided it; or as a Christian and see the Crucifixion as the actual voluntary surrender of all goodness into the hands of all evil, which somehow turns out to be a victory, *it is not reasonable*.

Paul, in 1 Corinthians, says that this crucified Messiah is an obstacle the Jews cannot get over, and to the Greeks is madness. Well, I have news for you, Paul: even after two thousand years of preaching a crucified Christ, there are a number of us devout *Christians* for whom the whole notion is not a piece of cake.

The cross is the cosmic focal point of the dilemma we Christians have created; it makes crystal clear the corner into which we have painted ourselves. We might have opted for an onmipotent God or we might have opted for an all-loving one. But we, in the face of overwhelming evidence to the contrary, have refused to settle for less than both. This, then, is the precise formulation of the prime Christian koan: an all-loving, all-powerful God either allows or causes evil and suffering in the world. You might call our unwillingness to let go of either horn of our dilemma theistic greed. And theologians ever since have been engaged in an enterprise known as theodicy—the attempt to save harmless, hold blameless, and vindicate the all-powerful, all-loving, all-just God we proclaim in the face of all the evil among us, not to mention the widespread suffering caused by disease and what are ironically singled out to be called acts of God.[4]

Lest this notion rise like a helium balloon and become an abstract (and safe) exercise in theological speculation, I should like to offer two things to help keep it quite earthy for us. The first is a story, and the second is a spiritual exercise almost guaranteed to help you make the dilemma of theodicy your very own.

### Bring on the Pain

This is a story about letting go into pain. Early in my practice of psychotherapy, a very abusive, assaultive, disdainful, and withholding patient was referred to me. It would be gross understatement to say that our hours together were no fun: they were for me excruciating and lonely. I dreaded those sessions and spent them in a defensive and exhausting self-protective posture.

Perhaps a snippet from our dialogue would help you understand how I felt:

"I tell you how stupid my boss is and you sit there! You are such a dork!"

(Silence)

"Oh! The silent treatment? Terrific. Is that what they taught you in 'shrink school?' "

"You can't fathom that my silence might be

neither punitive nor personal. Maybe I just have nothing useful to say right now.''

"Right *now*? Hell, man, you haven't said anything useful for eight months. You know, I haven't got a clue why I keep coming back here twice a week. I think it's turned into a bad habit, you know, like picking your nose.''

"Picking your nose would be a hell of a lot cheaper.''

"Oh, great. Now I get wise-ass remarks.''

Two hours of this every week, pretty much nonstop from start to finish. My responses frequently were ''wise-ass remarks.'' Increasingly so. It was my fumbling way of trying to protect myself from the abuse. Finally, I brought the matter up with my clinical supervisor, who borrows much from Eastern thought and spiritual practice in his psychotherapeutic and supervisory technique. His advice to me was unambiguous and firm: "You're absolutely right!'' he said. "You shouldn't trust this guy for at least four years.'' It was exactly what I wanted to hear.

What happened to the therapy, of course, was that it went to hell in a handbasket. Defended as I was (now with permission), absolutely *nothing* happened between the patient and me. I went back to my supervisor, perplexed. "I suspect you're not being careful enough,'' he offered. "Apparently, he's still getting to you. You'll have to burrow in deeper.'' So I did.

My remarks got even more acerbic, my interpretations cold and hostile. The nastier he got, the stingier I got. And vice versa. Several weeks of this routine brought the therapy almost to collapse. It seemed certain that the patient was going to quit. In one last desperate attempt to save it, I pushed my mentor's advice to its limits. The patient came in and I resolutely withheld *everything*. I said not one word for the entire hour. It was dreadful. But toward the end of the hour, as I sat there, absolutely safe (if totally ineffectual) and listened to this fellow's disdainful, hate-filled diatribe, mostly directed at me, the lightbulb went on. "None of this has a damn thing to do with *me*," I thought, "so what the hell am I defending?"

I went back to my mentor, furious. "I can't do this for four years!" I screamed. He started to snort and chuckle. "He's just attacking his own shadows, isn't he?" I shouted. My supervisor let go with a belly-ripping guffaw. "You can laugh," I protested, "but if I don't get in there and name this stuff, he's going to fire me and with good cause!" At this point, my mentor practically rolled on the floor in riotous convulsions. Then, shifting moods almost instantaneously and assuming a wistful demeanor, he eyed me ruefully and added, "Of course, it's going to be long, lonely, painful work. You've got to just straightforwardly name his stuff time and time again. Just a clear mirror. No defensiveness. No revenge. That's all your stuff and you've got to keep it out of the room." "Yeah, I know," I said quietly, with enormous resignation. Then sternly he rejoined, "So what do you think you're getting paid for? A joy ride?"

What a relief! But it was absolutely necessary to me to have pushed my resistance to its limits before I could simply let go and do the painful work required to help this very stuck patient.

And you, too, each of you for whom AIDS has become a part of your life, whether as one afflicted or as an involved bystander, must do the same. You must drink the bitter cup to its dregs and gag, sputter, spit, and swear if you ever hope to reach serenity with this disease.

### Practicing Theodicity

Now for the spiritual exercise designed to help you know theodicy personally. All you will need for this is the short phrase, "Here is God." The idea is to get that phrase going in your head like an Eastern mantra: "Here is God. Here is God. Here is God." If you are intent on doing this well, I would advise you to try to keep it going for a whole day.

Now sometimes, the words will come very easily—like when you have some pious thought, or it is a lovely day, or something wonderful has happened in the world. Yes, at those sweet moments, the warm fuzzies of religious sentiment will enfold you like so many delightful cirrus clouds.

But now try your mantra when you pass a rat-infested abandoned lot in a slum; or have some murderous, hateful thought; or read about the latest terrorist attack; or hear on the news about the most recent rape in your city or about another natural disaster. Now watch the warm fuzzies turn into cold pricklies.

In the past year, for instance, you might consider that we have witnessed an earthquake that killed twenty thousand more or less innocent men, women, and children, leaving behind tens of thousands more in numb agony, many of whom will never recover psychologically from the horror of the experience. We have witnessed also several thousand South Africans brutally murdered for the sake of preserving white supremacy. We have seen in Central America several more thousand of God's children sacrificed to the god of United States "security." Now try your mantra: Here is God?

Since this book is about the spiritual dilemma of AIDS, let us drive ourselves a little further into the morass of this paradox by looking at the pain this particular disease creates.

First, there is the pain of those who actually *have* AIDS. The ongoing physical wasting caused by the disease would be hard enough for a person with AIDS to endure. Many lose almost half their body weight before dying (six-foot tall, formerly strapping young men withering to eighty pounds). And then there is the not-uncommon dementia—the slow Alzheimer's-like erosion of the brain resulting in personality deterioration, loss of control of bodily functions, and finally death, as neurological control of vital organs is lost. It is hard to imagine the experience of this happening to your perhaps once-lithe body and acute mind. For starters, it must be terrifying. Try your mantra again now. Oh yes, I insist: Here is God, the all-loving One.

But there is a host of opportunistic diseases and symptoms associated with AIDS as well, each with its own pains: the disfiguring lesions of Kaposi's sarcoma all over and inside one's body; the suffocation (sometimes to death) of pneumocystis carinii; the thick white coating inside one's mouth caused by thrush; the repeated, sometimes nightly, drenching sweats and high fevers; the perpetual diarrhea; and then all the complications arising from these ailments or combinations thereof.

Besides the physical and mental anguish of having these things happen to you and the pain of the treatments used to try to cure the opportunistic diseases (radiation and chemotherapies, for example), there is also the hopelessness of the disease. Of the people diagnosed in 1981, 96 percent are now dead. This is (despite the occasional report of a miraculous recovery) a very fatal disease. It may be months or years before you die (five years at most), but die you will, probably after repeated bouts of opportunistic diseases. And your dying probably will not be easy. No matter how good you are to your body, no matter what treatment you undergo, this is almost assuredly a "one strike and you're out" disease; there appear to be no second chances. Time again for . . . Is God really *here*, do you think? The all-powerful One?

But this is not the end of the mental anguish for those afflicted with AIDS. As if dealing with the disease itself were not enough, there is the reaction of onlookers. Abandonment of gay PWA's by lovers, families, and friends is commonplace. In many locations, a gay PWA also has to endure the revulsion and neglect of hospital workers.[5] Imagine also, from your hospital bed, or if you are out of the hospital at the moment, at home, having to hear on your television and radio, or to read in newspapers and magazines, or to hear on the street that some people think you, a gay person with AIDS, deserve it. This can take the form of a Jerry Falwell calling this disease "retribution from God"; or of a teenage kid, insecure about his manhood, harassing you, a "fag," about AIDS as a way to reassure himself of his potency; or it can even take the form in the gay community of a callous judgmentalism. I heard a gay man recently say of a twenty-two-year-old boy dying at that very moment in the hospital, "Oh, he was just a little whore." These are all cases of blaming the victim as a way to avoid owning the pain of the disease. But at what price to the afflicted? How's the mantra going?

But perhaps the deepest and hardest-to-handle piece of anguish a gay PWA must face is his own reaction to such abuse. How many, having been told all their lives that they are sinful or sick or disgusting by virtue of their being gay, actually deep down believe that they deserve this disease?

A young man I never knew, but whose father shared his son's diary with me after he had died, wrote as his last legible entry (before the dementia made the final page incoherent), "I am an abomination against God. I am going to hell. And I deserve [it]."

Where did this come from? Though his parents were not of a fundamentalist stripe, the seeds of such feelings probably were very old. But I also happen to know that the hospital in which the young man died had on staff as chaplain an evangelical minister who began every first encounter with a gay AIDS patient with this harangue: "Friend, God has brought this disease on you because of the sinful, perverted life you have led! You are despicable to God! You are an abomination! This disease is God's just punishment on you for your terrible sinfulness. Now, you're going to die, friend. You hear me? DIE! SO, unless you want to endure the everlasting fires of hell, I urge you to *change your ways,* repent right now, and ask the Lord for forgiveness so that you at least have a chance of heaven, even if it is slim. What do you say?"

Would that those who desecrate the Good News in so gross a fashion could really taste the anguish in that boy's final words. The self-righteous, misguided chaplain in question placed a vulnerable, dying, demented young man in an untenable situation: he demanded that the boy change his *ontology,* his actual constitution. The young man knew he could not do that. (How many studies will it require to convince these fervent, self-righteous rigorists whose prejudice deafens them to facts that a gay person's sexuality is as given and unnegotiable as that of a straight person?) The young man's only alternative then—since he apparently believed the preacher—was to accept the sentence. I don't know about you, but the words "Here is God" just plain stick in my throat when confronted with this one.

Almost all that has just been said could probably also be said of PWAs who contract AIDS through the sharing of needles while illegally using drugs, although I suspect in our society that there is less stigma attached to a drug abuser than to a gay person. Drug abuse, after all, is still classified as a mental disorder—these people are perceived as sick, addicted. In most people's eyes, however, gay folks (no longer classified by the American Psychiatric Association as mentally ill by virtue of being homosexual)[6] now can only be labeled depraved.

But what of the blood product recipients who have done nothing more than need blood and as a result have contracted AIDS? And what of the children with AIDS? Here again, the societal terror of death has led to grossly irrational behavior around these victims and added anguish for them. Even though medical studies have proved that families with children who have AIDS—after five years of sharing toilets, eating and drinking utensils, and physical affection—are absolutely free of the disease, even though a sibling or parent has never contracted the disease from a child with AIDS living at home, nevertheless panic leads whole communities to oust children with AIDS from schools and recreational facilities, depriving these dying kids of the company and comfort of their friends at a time when they most need them. Is God's presence obvious to you here?

But what of us bystanders, near and far? Again let us begin with the gay context. First, there are the lovers of AIDS victims who not only must deal with the loss of their perhaps-lifelong mates, but also with the possibility of having contracted the disease themselves. In the midst of their grieving, they also frequently are excluded from wakes, funerals, and the comfort of shared bereavement afforded the families of their former lovers. Then there is the terror of those who get ill but not quite ill enough to be given the actual AIDS diagnosis—the terror of waiting for the other foot to fall. And then there are those of us who have lost friends, sometimes dozens of them, sometimes best friends, while we hear on the street new jokes like, "Know what the letters G-A-Y stand for? Got AIDS Yet?" It is hard to live surrounded by such hate.

There are also the families of gay AIDS victims. Frequently, their finding out about their son's AIDS is also the first time parents hear about his gayness. This is excruciating, especially since in many situations the PWA is too sick or demented by that point to be able to help his parents work through all their feelings about having a gay son, let alone a *dying* gay son.

A married couple of my acquaintance was informed by an attending physician of their son Tim's AIDS only when the young man was to be discharged from the hospital and had no place to go. Tim had asked the physician not to tell them. The doctor, in good conscience, could not comply. He was desperate. Having no place to send Tim to live, he felt it worth the risk to ask his mother and father. "Mr. and Mrs. R., your son has AIDS and is dying. There is no more we can do in the hospital. I need to find a place for him to stay. Do you have any suggestions?" They were good people and, after a stunned silence, immediately if weakly answered, "Well, of course he'll come live with *us*. He will come *home*."

They were simple folks. They hardly understood AIDS, let alone homosexuality. By the time he got home, Tim's mind was so deteriorated that he could hardly recognize his parents, let alone explain things to them. His condominium had to be vacated. In cleaning out his things, they found enough evidence to know for sure that their dying, demented son was gay. Sadly, no one helped them work through all of this before he died. I have since spent about ten hours with them, not only as a psychotherapist, but also as a kind of surrogate gay son, someone with whom they can try, by proxy, to make the kind of peace they never had the chance to make with Tim. But how many parents of gay sons in this predicament *never* get the chance?

What of the pain of parents of drug-abusing children? How much guilt has been experienced through predictable responses like "If I had been a better parent . . . "? How much self-loathing must drug-abusing mothers feel who have given the disease to their children in utero? What of parents of blood recipient children who have to watch their son or daughter not only die but be shunned by friends and excluded from school? How many such parents are, in turn, also shunned by irrationally terrorized people who assume that the parents of the child must also be infected now, too?

And on the broadest possible scale, one must not overlook the pain and confusion of all of us caught off guard by this disease. It is true, we were not prepared for mortality to break into our midst so brutally. And it is true that we played some role in getting ourselves into this situation. But death denial was well underway long before the current generation—subtly, surreptitiously. We are as much victims of it as perpetuators. It *is* terrifying. The pain we experience at the breaking of death into our midst is quite real.

There have been, as of this writing, about 21,000 people diagnosed with AIDS in the United States. By the year 1991, there will be 250,000 or more. The hope of finding a treatment and a vaccine for AIDS is slim. First, this is a "retrovirus," a virus whose RNA apparently "reeducates" the DNA in its host cell to make more virus. Apparently, no cure for a retrovirus infection has ever been developed.[7] Furthermore, this virus mutates rapidly, not only between people, but in the *same* person over the course of his illness. How in God's name do you create a vaccine against an ever-changing antigen?

Well, do you still have your mantra going? "Here is God. Here is God." Can you say it in the midst of all this agony? "Here is God. Here is God whose merciful love is without end. Here is God the omnipotent." Does it not give you pause? Does it not tie your stomach into knots? Does it not push your faith to its limits? Do you perhaps feel an urge at this point to shake your fist at heaven? To follow Abraham's or Job's lead and chastise God for this seeming sadistic treatment of His creatures? Would you perhaps even curse Her?

Maybe your faith is deeper than mine. Maybe this is not your response at all. But I must claim this reaction as mine, at least some of the time. Because, you see, the bad news is that AIDS truly *does* make no sense—all this pain, all this crucifixion among us. There is no solution to this or any other koan. No theologian has yet synthesized a successful theodicy; none has ever developed a logic that makes God seem truly just in the light of the kind of pain AIDS causes. There is no easy way out of this dilemma.

Rabbi Harold Kushner, author of the popular book *When Bad Things Happen to Good People*,[8] in trying to make peace with his young son's death, opted for a belief in a good but *not* all-powerful God, a God who has no control over nature. It is tempting, but I just cannot bite. That's only half a God, in my book.

And a not all-good God I want no part of.

There is no solution to the paradox theodicy attempts to solve. And that, in fact, is the orthodox Christian position about it: we simply *cannot* know the why of evil and pain in the world in light of our belief in God's limitless love and power. So what now? What now?

### Out of Despair, a Response

When I reach this point in my AIDS contemplation, I always find myself at the edge of despair. I am helpless against this vile disease. And I am powerless before the God who either inflicts or permits it. What is worse, I can make no sense of it. For me, perhaps the most repulsive, unconscionable image is of a fetus infected with AIDS. Dear God, why? To what end? I want to primally scream heavenward, "HOW CAN YOU DO THIS!"

Then the tears come. Copiously, often enough. For all my friends who are dead. For those suffering. For the frightened as well. For all the hatred this miserable plague has evoked.

And with the flow of tears comes also the release of the knot at the pit of my stomach. Quieter tears now. And in that subdued, defeated moment, when out of sheer exhaustion I abandon my ultimate dependence on reason, as I sit and weep for all the anguish of AIDS in our lives, letting myself free-fall now into the pain of it, its quality changes. Oh, it still hurts. But it is now a sparkling pain, an energizing pain, a purging pain.

And in the relief of my yielding, I come to know that the ancient spiritual epithet is true that says, "Power is in the yielding." Because with my surrender comes a rush of energy and almost, strangely enough, joy. Just at the moment when it seems there is nothing to be done—that all is hopeless—at that very moment I become charged with vitality and the will to do everything that needs to be done. More than the flesh will allow.

And that, my brothers and sisters, is, I am convinced, the *key* to bearing the pain of this awful ordeal. While there is no answer to Job, or to the survivors of the Colombian earthquake, or to the dead in Northern Ireland, or to the twenty thousand men, women, and children who are expected to contract AIDS this year; while there is no *answer* that will relieve the pain, nothing to do right now that will make AIDS go away; there is, as suggested at the end of the last chapter, a *response* that will make it all bearable: it is to love.

The disciples asked Jesus, "Who sinned, this man or his parents, that he was born blind?" (John 9:2). Jesus replied, "It was not that this man sinned, or his parents, but that the works of God might be made manifest in him." And then He *tended to the man.* In a symbolic gesture of human-divine compassion, He stooped down, made some mud with His own spit, spread it on the man's eyes, and miraculously restored his sight.

If the disciples had asked our Lord, "Who sinned, this man or his parents, that he has AIDS?" what do you think Jesus would have replied? How do you think He would have responded? Do you think He would have blamed the victim, as Mr. Falwell seems smugly content to do? I think not. I believe Jesus' reply would have been exactly the same as His original one: "It was not that this man sinned, or his parents, but that the works of God might be made manifest in him." And I also have no doubt that with human-divine compassion He would then have healed the man.

We most often have heard this lesson to mean that in order to reveal Jesus' divinity—His divine healing power—God made the man blind. But this is to miss a simpler and broader meaning. You see, *each* of us has as much power as Jesus had to tend to that blind man. We might not be able to restore his sight, but that is inconsequential. The point is that while we cannot know *why* pain exists, the only response that can redeem it—make it life-giving rather than life-draining—is our surrender to it and our tending to the needs of the afflicted.

Here, practically, there usually must be a parting of ways—a division of labor, if you will. For it is mostly the work of those dying to surrender, and mostly the work of bystanders lovingly to look after those in pain. C. S. Lewis, in his book *The Problem of Pain*,[9] describes the situation thus: "What is good in any painful experience is, for the sufferer, his submission to the will of God, and, for the spectators, the compassion aroused and the acts of mercy to which it leads."

In fact, this is too pat a distinction. I have been awed by the enormous outpouring of love I have witnessed in some of my dying gay brothers. These were—and are—men who not only made peace with their dying, but were free enough—in the midst of their loss—to help others who were afflicted come to a peaceful place, and even to reach out to the rest of the gay community to help them also grow through this experience.

Nevertheless, giving up to the pain of having AIDS and making peace with impending death are the principal works PWAs must be about. And the first half of this chapter was mostly for them. Oh, do it passionately, my brothers and sisters. It is the only way through. Tap the deepest, darkest recesses of your rage and despair.

## On Going Down Fighting

In this regard, something more needs to be said about those people who seem to go down fighting. I remember a story a priest I know included in a sermon she preached shortly after her father had died.[10] He had died of emphysema. His last few days, mostly comatose, included his having repeatedly to heave to get enough air—wrenching, belly-ripping gasps, one after the other. This woman's initial response was to feel, "Oh, let go, daddy. You don't need to keep doing this. Let go. Please let go." It was so painful, you see, for her to watch him in such agony.

Then as she sat by his deathbed for several days, watching him heave and gasp, and had no choice but to get used to it, she had time to recall how much her father had loved living, how much he had cherished the vineyard he had planted and tended, and what hunger he had had for all life offered. And then she could appreciate that he was now doing exactly what was in character for him: he was getting every last breath he could. And so her response changed and she could be with him fully in his last hours, resonating with him, "Yes, *breathe,* daddy! Yes, that's it. One more! And now another!" This seems to me a perfectly worthy death, a death that had its own integrity, its own kind of surrender.

People with AIDS not infrequently, I observe, go down fighting. And this poses a problem in terms of a current mindset about dying that merits attention.

The most widespread way of approaching death for the past twenty years, at least among the helping professions, has relied on the model developed by Elisabeth Kübler-Ross.[11] It would seem an easy matter simply to extend the Kübler-Ross model to those dying with AIDS. And in fact, this has been done and has, to some extent, been helpful.

But I also think that AIDS has exposed the limitations of the Kübler-Ross model. This model gives us a wonderful, logical way of conceptualizing a person's response to his or her death—the passage from resistance (flight or fight) to acceptance (just being). This model (like all models) is of course *conceptual*. And lest we forget, Dr. Kübler-Ross's stages (denial, anger, bargaining, depression, and acceptance) were originally presented simply as states she *observed* in many dying patients.

Quickly enough, however, even in her own mind, this progression changed from being descriptive to being prescriptive. Acceptance came to be cherished as the best of all possible states to be in at the moment of death. And once that value was in place, you might say that the Kübler-Ross model turned into the "industry standard" for dying.

The problem is that acceptance came to be defined as a sort of placid, blissful, laid-back state of mind. But many AIDS patients simply do not die the Kübler-Ross way (and neither do lots of other people). As we have seen, upon achieving remission from some opportunistic disease, many PWAs launch back into life (as has my historian friend from the previous chapter) with zest and gusto. I find it of no use to call this denial, in any sense of the word. Or bargaining, for that matter.

For those of us reared on Kübler-Ross, then, what do we have? A bunch of bad deaths? But what does it mean to say, "He died *wrong?*" Is there a sort of perverse expectation that some poor bastard is going to have to do it over until he gets it right?

If the Kübler-Ross model is used with people who have AIDS, I believe it will need to be used judiciously. I also believe that the word *acceptance* needs to be very broadly defined. It must be taken to mean achieving equanimity with both the external realities of the person's life (he or she is going to die) and with the internal realities (his or her personality). So, my brothers and sisters with AIDS, if you have been a fighter all your life, I suspect you will quite naturally go down with your dukes up. It seems an OK way to do it in my book. Have at it, I say.

I would share one further idea about the notion of surrender if you have AIDS. At a recent conference, a chaplain asked me what I thought patients should do who got angry with God. My response was, "They should tell the Bastard off!" OK. It was a glib one-liner. But I also meant it in earnest.

I have no compunction about expressing rage at God. In fact, I believe it is both crucial and a time-honored tradition. Almost every Jewish patriarch took God on.[12] St. Peter argued with Jesus about having his feet washed.[13] Even the pious St. Teresa of Avila, having been dumped off the back of a cart into the mud, picked herself up, looked furiously toward heaven, and chided, "No wonder you have so few friends! Look how you treat them!"

My advice is to offer to God all of your rage about your plight. Yell it at Him. Chastise Her, if that's what you feel. Call God whatever you need to in order to plumb the depths of your hurt and anger. And, for God's sake, don't feel guilty about it.

First of all, God can take it; She is not wounded by our rage. Moreover, I have no doubt God understands such rantings to be absolutely essential in order for us to reach equanimity with our pains and losses. In fact, I am persuaded that God swells with compassion at our angriest moments, aching with us in our rage. I am certain She wants to be with us at those explosive times. Call Him every name in the book if you must. It is a valid and worthy part of your spiritual work in dying.

The last word about expressing anger at God should come from Pierre Wolff who, in his book *May I Hate God?*, offers this powerful insight:

"When people express harsh feelings to the One or ones who are their object, love is *already* stronger in them than their feelings. Love is *already* transforming, transfiguring, this feeling into something else, something closer to love than to hatred. . . . Perhaps there is hatred present as long as people are mute, absolutely mute; but as soon as they decide to express what is in their heart to the other, something is *already* changing and maybe even *already* changed."[14]

### The Least Tincture of the Love of God

Now for the rest of us. In the preface to *The Problem of Pain*, C. S. Lewis humbly states that all he has to offer his readers is his conviction "that when pain is to be borne, a little courage helps more than much knowledge, a little human sympathy more than much courage, and the least tincture of the love of God more than all."[15] It is principally the task of those of us without AIDS to provide human sympathy and to be vehicles of God's love for those afflicted. And in the act of responding, I believe we too shall find comfort amid this nightmare.

In his book *Sister Death*,[16] O'Kelley Whitaker reminds us that dying people have four major concerns: first, that they will be as free of pain as possible; second, that they will die with dignity and not grotesquely; third, that they will die with loving friends around them; and finally, that they will find some answer to the question, What happens to me when I die?

I should think every single Christian could contribute something of his or her time or resources to ensure that those needs are met for every single PWA. There is nothing magical required, no special technical skill.[17] Were you at a dying man's bedside and the painkillers had reached their limit, and were he still in pain and feverish, would it require much of you simply to put a cool compress on his head? To add just that much more relief from the pain?

Would it require special training for you to visit a person with AIDS who might well be feeling grotesque—emaciated, with lesions from head to foot and tied to every kind of machine—and just to chat, helping him or her know the human dignity that transcends any physical deterioration?

Would you need to be a specialist to befriend a gay man who had been abandoned by everyone he knew to die in some antiseptic ward? It would require only asking the ward nurse which patient never had visitors.

And could not any compassionate person listen and be supportive as someone attempted to answer for herself those frightening questions about being and death?

There is nothing magical required of us. Almost every hospital and every gay clinic I know of has volunteer programs specially designed for AIDS wards.

What will you do?

I do not urge such loving care only because it is required of us as Christians. I urge it because I assume you picked up this book to try to achieve some spiritual peace with AIDS. In that case, the giving I advocate is crucial. Because it is my conviction that when we stop trying to blame the victim and when we give up trying to make God's ways seem humanly reasonable, then it is precisely through our acts of loving—of tending the sick and dying, of comforting the bereaved, and of striving to find a cure—that we spiritually feed and heal one another *and so bring in the kingdom*. Loving—loving as a verb, the act of loving—is the only way I know to bear the pain. In fact, I am convinced in the doing of it, we shall find that charity in the midst of incomprehensible anguish is its own and sufficient comfort.

# CHAPTER 5

# A Case for Heaven

It would be unconscionable for a Christian to write a book about a fatal illness without discussing heaven. And yet, how can one write about heaven in the late 1980s?

I can find no way through this morass without exploring what may be intricate (and for some, tedious) philosophical and theological territory. I ask your forebearance. For it is crucial that we solve this heaven-talk dilemma.

## *Heaven Talk and the Post-Enlightenment Mind*

As with most dilemmas, we are presented with two horns. On one horn, the question becomes, How does one say anything about heaven that will not alienate the skeptical, scientific, twentieth-century mind and make the whole enterprise seem foolish? This half of the quandary C.S. Lewis summed up in 1940 when he wrote:[1]

We are very shy nowadays of even mentioning heaven. We are afraid of the jeer about "pie in the sky" and of being told that we are trying to "escape" from the duty of making a happy world here and now into dreams of a happy world elsewhere. But either there is "pie in the sky" or there is not. If there is not, then Christianity is false, for this doctrine is woven into its whole fabric. If there is [pie in the sky], then this truth, like any other, must be faced, whether it is useful at political meetings or no.

The post-Enlightenment mind has no time for traditional talk of heaven as a reality. Since most Western intelligentsia have now placed Christianity on an equal footing with all other world religions, relegating it thus to the domain of anthropology, it is no longer of essential relevance. The whole eschatological realm has been recast in psychological terms: most educated Westerners would simply say that talk of heaven is rich symbolic language—primitive, if occasionally elegant, projection into the universe of the landscape of the unconscious mind. In everyday parlance, heaven is seen as a figment of our imaginations.

Ethics may be tolerably associated with religion. Inculcation of values seems by some appropriately placed at the Church's doorstep, although for others, school systems are the preferred agencies for training in this area.

Aesthetics are also considered appropriate to the religious endeavor. A recent survey conducted in a High Anglican parish included a list of possible reasons why the parishioner completing the questionnaire chose this particular congregation. "The music program" was the unchallenged winner (and indeed the parish's music program is lavish); "to worship God" came in third. One must at least commend the candor.

Social interaction is also an acceptable *raison d'être* for the Church in the late 1980s, although this usually does not connote any profound commitment

to community. Mostly, it implies socializing in the
most synthetic meaning of the word. Among intelligent, educated, nonsuperstitious Westerners, if the
Sunday morning ritual is not coffee and the *New York
Times* on the balcony, church is attended as a source
of inspiring talks about goodness; a place of antiquar-
ian and artistic preservation, and a nice place to meet
people, "worship" being, for many, a way to rev up
for coffee hour. And perhaps my own denomination—the Episcopal church—the best-educated (if
perhaps not the wealthiest) mainline denomination—
has some pre-eminence in fostering this state of
affairs.

But let us not be deceived that even *this* is the majority opinion. More than 60 percent of the population of the United States does not darken the door of a
church on any given Sunday, and even so, we Americans are a remarkably churchgoing bunch. In western
Europe (Ireland excepted), less than 10 percent of
the population attend church on any regular basis.

How, then, can one talk seriously of heaven to a
population that largely views the whole notion as an
ancient myth? This is one half of the problem.

### Heaven Talk and the Fundamentalist Mind

The other horn of the heaven-talk dilemma has to
do with the danger of perpetuating "Sunday school
religion" for adults. In point of fact, C.S. Lewis's
choice of words makes obvious the problem. Even *I*,
who believe that heaven talk is far from nonsense,
cringe at the words, "Either there is pie in the sky or

there is not." I find the notion of a pie-in-the-sky heaven as embarrassing and silly and repugnant as would the most thoroughgoing atheist.

In the United States especially, there is on the rise a ripple of piety that stands in reaction to the neutered, demythologized hulk of Christianity that mainline Christendom—a religion mostly devoid of any credible affirmation of supernatural truth—embodies. The new movement has opted for a radical and intentional regression to a more primitive consciousness. The fundamentalist-evangelical-born-again movement in Christianity, in its attempt to go back to some pure past—one untainted and uncorrupted by the twentieth century—demands of its followers that they put aside all of the evolved consciousness for which humanity has been groaning forward lo these two hundred years, and eschew many of the facts of science uncovered in that same period. Instead, this group is committed to "old-time religion." And this means, for most of its adherents, taking at face value (that is, literally) every word of the Bible, giving no real cognizance to the sociocultural or historical context out of which those words arose.

This, in effect, creates religion in a vacuum. Its adherents begin by assuming that Scripture is to be studied only on its own terms, ignoring the implicit cultural meaning of words themselves, the unavoidable editing produced by redaction and translation. They choose instead to believe that by some magic of accurate word-for-word translation (which in itself begs the question of interpretation), they truly have and hold in their hands the actual words of God that the Deity dictated to (inspired) human scribes who apparently were no more than accomplished stenographers.

Nor do grays exist in this fundamentalist universe. People are either good or bad; acts are either worthy or abominable; world events reflect either God's blessing or God's curse. No nuances are permitted in this cosmos: they would be too messy, too much of a bother.

This religious development is akin to creating a cult of Grimm's fairy tales. It perpetuates what I have called "Sunday school religion," a religion in which poetic images and illustrative religious stories are taken for real, a context in which things are made to appear simpler than they are. This approach is, of course, appropriate for children.

It is psychologically necessary for children that the world be kept less complex than it really is. The young are unable to take in and cope with the full blast of reality, especially in the twentieth century. A child needs a universe in which he or she feels safe, a circumscribed world in which someone will be there to protect, to nurture, to save from all harm. A child also needs things to be simple in the moral realm. There have to be bad guys and good guys, villains and heroes, Lex Luthor and Superman, the Wicked Witch of the West and Glinda. Children who are forced to deal too early with the full brunt of the world reach adulthood badly damaged, distrustful, unable to risk.

In the religious realm, children need the same kind of simplified world. They are not yet able to grasp abstract theological concepts; their cognitive powers are too inchoate for that. Try to help a child comprehend the Crucifixion. Or Incarnation. Or the Trinity. No, children need Noah's ark full of animals, really floating around, just like the story says. They need the primeval garden of Eden with a good God and a bad snake; the meek Jesus who puts children on his knee and dandles them; the good Joseph and his technicolor dreamcoat and his bad brothers. Moreover, religion for a child must be more emotional than cognitive; feelings are evolutionarily older and more available to children.

However, this new-wave conservative wing of Protestantism would, it seems, insist that this childlike world is the *real* world. It is, as I have said, rather like a sect that claims the scriptures contained in Grimm's tales are factual and definitive for life. If one wonders how any sentient person in the twentieth century with even a high school education could swallow such pap, I think it is easily comprehensible if one views the phenomenon as a poignant statement of the spiritual hunger of our age. Here is a group of relatively intelligent, educated people who are so disillusioned with the vapidity of antisepticized Christianity that most denominations dole out, and so starved for an affirmation of the supernatural dimension of reality, that they are prepared willingly to suspend their own cognitive sophistication and regress into a childlike state of consciousness in order to get fed.

It is not that I do not share their hunger, but there must be a better option. To begin with, such folks are *not* fed. They may *feel* fed, but it is as though they had ingested a diet of pure fiber: there is the sensation of fullness but with no nutritive intake. Lest this be challenged, I would point out that if "by their fruits ye shall know them," then the self-righteous, condescending condemnation spewed forth often enough by members of these sects upon those who do not buy their product, coupled with their seeming obliviousness to the plight of the poor, provide conclusive evidence to me that divine love beyond measure is *not* what they are being fed Sunday mornings.

There must be a better option, because this is too complicated and dangerous a world for consciousnesses formed only by Sunday school fairy tales. This is a world of few blacks and whites, and many grays. Adults need a religion that helps them develop a spirituality for the real world, the real twentieth-century world replete with its breathtaking speed of change, the horror of its starving masses, its practically incomprehensible and convoluted economics, and the terrifying game of brinkmanship nations seem willing to engage in, using nuclear weaponry as board pieces. And now it needs a spirituality to respond to a plague among us, just when we thought the earth had seen its last.

How are we to negotiate these tricky waters? More specifically, how are we, as real twentieth-century people, to discuss heaven, caught as we are between this Scylla and this Charybdis of scientism and fairy-tale religiosity?

### The Language Barrier

The dilemma is made doubly difficult because of language. Things spiritual cannot be adequately approached through logical discourse. Entry into the spiritual realm must usually be more aesthetic than cognitive. I am reminded of a delightful quotation on this matter from H. L. Mencken. "A solemn high mass must be a thousand times as impressive, to a man with any genuine religious sense in him, as the most powerful sermon ever roared under the big-top by a Presbyterian auctioneer of God. In the face of such overwhelming beauty it is not necessary to belabor the faithful with logic; they are better convinced by letting them alone."[2]

In our age, this need for the aesthetic in religious language results in making skewering on either horn of our dilemma practically unavoidable. It is all too easy to begin with the metaphors of Scripture pertaining to heaven, ride that wave into the glorious exploitation of those metaphors by the likes of Dante and Milton, and end up with religion as an appreciation of literature. (A professor of Bible [!] at the Divinity School of the University of Chicago seems to approach Scripture on just those terms.) This, of course, is no longer to be engaged in religion at all; it is rather to pursue comparative lit.

On the other hand, one can take those self-same metaphors of Scripture, use them to evoke pentecostal fervor, and then, from this experience of controlled hysteria, begin to behave as though the metaphors were facts. A forty-five-year-old Greek woman I know insists quite adamantly that God is an old man with a long white beard who wears shiny white robes and sits on a big throne on a cloud. (When I coyly suggest to her that God is *really* a black handicapped woman who is lesbian, she approaches catatonia.)

So one is faced with the dilemma of what kind of language to use in speaking of heaven today. All the best metaphors have been capitalized on, bastardized, trivialized, or beaten to death. I believe the solution to our dilemma will come from the least likely source.

### Toward a Solution: The Quantum

My undergraduate major was philosophy. Perhaps the most spiritually important course I took during those years was in the philosophy of science. In all candor, I hardly remember anything of the course's content (and it has been twenty years). But I remember walking away from that semester's endeavor both shocked and liberated. Shocked because (as also happens with first-year Scripture students) I had had a holy cow dethroned. In my case, it was our modern-day science-god who bit the dust. And liberated because this development once again allowed God to be God for me, and science to be exposed for the fake god it had been and, for many, still is.

There are two matters of scientific fact that I would like to present. The first is the assumption in science of causality. All scientific inquiry assumes some sequence in which A causes B. Chemical A reacts with chemical B to produce C. An object moving at a force X, upon striking a stationary object Y, will . . . There is scarcely a scientific pursuit that does not assume causality as a *law*—that is, as always true. And this "fact" of science pervades every practical application of it right down to the expectation that when you depress the handle on your toaster, the current will flow through the heating coils and subject your English muffin to a slow burn.

But causality, in point of fact, cannot be proved. One can combine chemicals A and B a thousand thousand times and each time produce C. Each time, the *probability* of causality is reinforced. But there is no proof that on the one millionth, one hundred thousandth, four hundred and sixty-third try, it will *not* produce Z. Causality cannot be proved by any amount of empirical data. In fact, it cannot be proved by any known means at all. Please pause for a moment and contemplate that a cornerstone of scientific pursuit and all modern technology rests on an unproved, unprovable assumption.

We behave as though causality were fact, simply because it has been reconfirmed often enough for us in everyday life that we trust it. In other words, for practical purposes, it is useful to assume the principle of causality. It is also psychologically attractive since it gives us the comforting illusion of predictability in a fast-changing world. But causality is, in a sense, a convenient fiction. We have chosen to treat it as proved, but in the *real* world—the world in its fullness—the universal principle of causality is unsubstantiated.

In point of fact, in the past thirty years, based upon observations made possible by quantum mechanics and electron microscopy, scientists have had to admit into their universe the fact of unpredictability. Physicist Gary Zukav, in *The Dancing Wu Li Masters*, summarizes it in this way: "Given a beam of electrons, quantum theory can predict the probable distribution of the electrons over a given space at a given time, but quantum theory cannot predict, *even in principle*, the course of a single electron."[3] Zukav concludes this discussion by stating, "The whole idea of a causal universe is undermined by the uncertainty principle."

"Uncertainty principle" was the name given to Heisenberg's discovery that there is no way to observe something without the observer changing that which is observed.[4] In particular, there is no known way (and assumed to be no way at all) to observe an electron without altering it. In Heisenberg's own words, published in the *Zeitschrift für Physik* in 1927, "We *cannot* know, as a matter of principle, the present in all its details."

Now I would like to observe two things about this principle. First, it is, I think, amusing that something whose essence is unpredictability has been named by the scientific community, a principle. It seems a very human, if pathetic, attempt to appear to be in control precisely of that which is out of control.

Second, shuffled off to the side as it is by the large majority of scientists who need to be about their empirical work and who haven't time for these minor exceptions, this uncertainty principle would appear to be relegated to the "minor curiosity" heap. But I would offer this as the stunning *denouement* of the myth of scientific objectivity. The unpredictability of electron movement of which we are speaking theoretically exists in every atom of the universe. One might well conclude, then, that uncertainty is the most prevalent basic fact of the universe. And one would be making this assertion based on empirical scientific evidence. Where is the universal principle of causality now?

I have presented this undoing of one of the commonly assumed "unshakable" pillars of science as a dramatic example. But, in fact, the same process could be undertaken with any of the principles of science. As Hans Küng has made amply clear in his book *Does God Exist?*[5], contemporary philosophers who explore theories of knowledge all seem to reach the same conclusion: knowing *anything* inevitably begins by assuming (believing) *something*. Küng quotes W. Stegmüller:[6] "We must not deny knowledge to make room for faith. Instead, we must believe something from the outset in order to be able to talk of knowledge or science at all."

As Küng then notes, "All knowledge thus contains a 'presupposition' that can be described as 'matter of faith.' " Quoting Stegmüller again, he adds, "The alternative usually understood as 'faith or reason,' implying the distinction between religious experience and scientific knowledge, is misleading."[7]

But it is precisely the widely accepted myth of the "hardness" of scientific knowledge versus the presumed "softness" of religious experience that has left Western civilization in such a sorry state of spiritual privation.

The other scientific matter that I would like us to consider involves our notions of the linearity of time and the Newtonian geometry of space. Before Einstein, time was assumed to be linear, and progressing everywhere the same throughout the universe. It all moved forward one cosmic tick at a time. And space was one enormous grid that could be measured out in meters or feet in all directions, neatly, squarely, to infinity. Again, all empirical data proved this to be true. Newton's laws were taken as descriptive, unassailable facts. Until $E = mc^2$. And now (after a wrenching scientific paradigm shift occasioned by the special theory of relativity) time and space are no longer considered linear. It is accepted that they are actually curved.

It is practically impossible to visualize curved time and space. As for time, it is most easily glimpsed by an example. If a man and his twin brother parted and the first took off in a space capsule and zoomed around the galaxy for a bit while his brother continued his humdrum earthly existence, after the first's reentry into the stratosphere and upon the joyful reunion of the two, those twin siblings would no longer be the same age. The man who had taken the intergalactic tour now would be calculably younger than his brother.

I don't know about you, but I find this development more than a little unnerving. Frankly, I find it awesome. And we must remember this notion is now accepted scientific *fact*; it is included within the working scientific paradigm of our age. The idea of curved space is for me beyond conceptualization; I simply cannot fathom it.

Again, it should be noted that civilization continues to behave as though linear time and regular geometry were realities. Why? Because they are useful fictions. The same kind of convenient obliviousness that most of the scientific world engages in vis-à-vis the pervasive uncertainty in the universe obtains here as well. We prefer to live with a fiction because in our circumscribed existence, life is easier if we do so. Or to state this psychologically, the world seems much more within our control this way. In fact, this was one of Einstein's greatest bugaboos. He mostly rejected quantum mechanics. And the depth of his resistance to admitting even possible uncertainty into his universe is reflected in his unflinching assertion, "God does not play dice!"

## From Quantum to Mystery

I have chosen these two matters of scientific discovery because they dramatically and clearly challenge the throne of our generally secure science-god. An accomplished philosopher of science or knowledge could undoubtedly present a more thorough, cogent, and better-illustrated case. For this bumbling attempt, I apologize.

Nevertheless, you might ask, what has all this to do with heaven? A great deal, I think. For you see, as J. B. Phillips reminded us in his book *Your God Is Too Small*[8], it is the job of any religion to preach only the broadest possible reality. Religion is false if it is not rooted in a cosmic context. The religious camera takes deceiving photographs unless its focal point is set to infinity. Religion must have as its stock-in-trade those things that are ultimately and cosmically true.

It has been empirically demonstrated by the scientific community that the most prevalent, pervasive characteristic of the universe is unpredictability and that time and space are curved. These are realities of enormous dimension, and hence, spiritual consequence.

First, we must clarify what it really means to say that something is unpredictable. To declare something uncertain or unpredictable is in fact to own that it is, to the observer, incomprehensible. Dwell on that for a moment: to say something cannot be predicted is to confess that it is beyond your ability to understand, that your way of comprehending and organizing reality does not work here.

The scientific community dislikes *not* comprehending. It likes even less not knowing how to comprehend that which it wishes to study. It does not like to admit that its matrix for observing reality misses things. Yet even John Gribbin, a noted physicist, in his book *In Search of Schrodinger's Cat*, states in support of the "many worlds" theory of the universe now espoused by numerous scientists:

The uncomfortable feature that has prevented this improved interpretation from taking the world of physics by storm is that it implies the existence of many other worlds—possibly an infinite number of them—existing in some way sideways across time from our reality.

This "many worlds" theory is described by Gribbin using the following metaphor proposed by the theory's originator, Hugh Everett:

I carry out an experiment in a closed room, then come out and tell you the result, which you tell a friend in New York, who reports it to someone else, and so on. At each step, the wave function becomes more complex, and embraces more of the "real world." But at each stage the alternatives remain equally valid, overlapping realities, until the news of the outcome of the experiment arrives. We can imagine the news spreading across the whole universe in this way, until the whole universe is in a state of overlapping wave functions, alternative realities that only collapse into one world when observed. But who observes the universe?[9]

Please remember, these are the words of a physicist, not a theologian.

In religious jargon, matters of this sort used to be called mysteries. So let us then draw this empirically substantiated, scientific conclusion: the most prevalent activity in the cosmos, apparently affecting every atom in existence, is shrouded in mystery. In its very uncertainty, the life of every atom bespeaks the boundless unknowability of the cosmos. The most powerful tools of microscopy and mathematics would seem to have brought about the wholesale demise of the monolithic unshakability of science. In the unpredictable quiverings of perhaps all cosmic matter, our objective, objectifiable science-god would seem to have castrated himself.

In light of this, one must ask the scientific intelligentsia of our age, "*Who* is living in illusion?" Which endeavor *truly* belongs in the cultural anthropology department: the discipline that claims the basic unknowability of God (which is only a way of affirming the ultimate mystery of the universe that the uncertainty principle confirms), or the endeavor that largely continues to follow the myth of universal causality? Which should be consigned to the archives as one more quaint attempt of primitive humankind to explain the frightening mysteries of the universe? Which has more the character of aboriginal religion?

I do not purport to be a scientist. But as a layman, my response to those quantum jumping electrons I once viewed in a film simulation of them was deeply religious. To be informed that I live in a universe reverberating with humanly incomprehensible energy was to hear reaffirmed that "the heavens are telling the glory of God" (Ps. 19:1). To have acknowledged that the movement of all matter, at its most microscopic level, dwells in inaccessible mystery was to be given permission to worship again a fathomless God "who has measured the waters in the hollow of [His] hands and marked off the heavens with a span, enclosed the dust of the earth in a measure and weighed the mountains in scales (Isa. 40:12). To grasp that this incomprehensible energy pervades the universe was to grasp anew that ". . . He is before all things, and by Him all things consist" (Col. 1:17).

In like manner, to glimpse curved time and curved space is to open myself to the reality of dimensions whose enormity I cannot conceive. If time was formerly believed to extend into an infinite past and an infinite future (concepts that were awesome enough), what does one do now with the idea of infinities of time that cosmically turn in on themselves in eternal helixes or circles or spheres? What does *now* mean now? It is no longer merely a point on a line; of that, we are assured. So does this current moment of curved time now simultaneously exist in

more than one temporal plane? What of the next moment? Does it at some cosmic intersection coexist
with the moment here present? What of that moment
(expressed in our archaic linear fashion) "after"
death? Am I then being in some moment in some other cycle of curved time in some location in the warp
of this no-longer regularly geometrical cosmos?

And if I take yet one more quantum leap and try to
fathom God's time and space, time and space ever-
curving, giving rise to ever-new incarnations of the
same-but-different matter in succeeding same-but-different moments, do time and space then merge into
one perduring moment of Being—never ceasing,
alive, scintillating cycles of being in which God's
mysterious energy fully consists?

Are we then reconciled with those ancient words,
"In Him, we live and move and have our being (Acts
17:28)"? Have we now heeded Paul's exhortation to
"look not at the things which are seen, but at the
things which are not seen: for the things which are
seen are temporal; but the things which are not seen
are eternal" (2 Cor. 4:18)?

Do not those ancient metaphors, whose writers'
consciousnesses could not have begun to conceptualize curved time or space or multiple worlds come incredibly close to grasping the truth of these apparent
realities? In light of these recent discoveries of modern science—if we stand honestly and vulnerably in
their presence—can we *help* but posit a kingdom not
of this world?

The honest answer, of course, is "yes, many could

and *do*." Many stand and gaze at these wonders and only shrug.

I am not contending that the truths of this new scientific paradigm *prove* the existence of either God or heaven. The Church has tried that tactic in the past using former paradigms and has ended up with egg on its face. The problem is that, as Marilyn Ferguson has exquisitely described in her book *The Aquarian Conspiracy*,[10] paradigms come and go, the incumbent sure to be overthrown by some later contender. It is, then, only a matter of time before the relativity paradigm is itself replaced.

But I *am* saying this: when we push our knowledge to its limit, regardless of which paradigm we accept as our context, we end up at *mystery*. I would also posit that each succeeding paradigm pushes us to broader and broader reaches of this mystery. It is one of Ferguson's most salient insights that paradigm shifts occur precisely because the new paradigm makes more meaningful a larger span of reality than was illuminated by its predecessor.

Nevertheless, when we reach this outer edge— however far it may be—and we empirically can know no more, we are faced with a choice: faith or meaninglessness. To give a specific application of this, either the mystery revealed by the uncertainty principle points to God or it points to cosmic absurdity. And if the latter be true, humanity has no escape from despair, because we would have to conclude that the most pervasive characteristic of the universe holds no meaning at all.

### Reclaiming Intuitive Knowledge

The secular world would call choosing belief in God at this point a leap of faith. But we have already debunked the false distinction between religious and scientific knowing. Both, as we have seen, begin with presuppositions (articles of faith). Küng demonstrates this with great clarity by describing the stance of the atheist.[11] "Denial of God implies an ultimately unjustified fundamental trust in reality . . . If someone denies God, he does not know why he ultimately trusts reality." And yet, it may justifiably be asked here, when faced with the mystery, why posit *God* or, in the context of this chapter, *heaven*?

I would suggest that the answer in part comes from acknowledging two fundamental kinds of human knowing, cognitive and intuitive. Carl Jung, in formulating his personality typology,[12] noted that we apprehend things in two ways and tend to be of one type or the other in this behavior: we are either intuitive (relying on sudden insights) or sensing (sensing here means relying on one's senses to take in the universe—that is, absorbing large quantities of data). Jung also differentiated between those of us who tend to think our way through in making decisions about things, and those of us who rely mostly on feelings. Science, it would seem, relies most heavily on apprehending things through the acquisition of data and on deciding about things by the use of logical thought. In Jungian terms, this is sensing-thinking behavior.

Conversely, other human pursuits, among them

religion, I would contend, rely mostly on intuition—the sudden "Aha!" experience—to apprehend things, and on feelings to decide about them. Again in Jungian terms, this would be intuitive-feeling behavior.

In our age, we have tended to discount the intuitive-feeling kind of knowing as somewhat bogus. At best, it is seen as the handmaid of scientific thought; at worst, useful only for amusement. The ascendancy of science has enthroned sensing-thinking knowledge as "the real thing." The world runs on it these days; it has built skyscrapers and electroencephalographs—it has proved itself. The other kind of knowing, judged as insubstantial bordering or frivolous, is feared to lead to dissolution (Marx's opium theory; Freud's illusion theory).

But this is a great impoverishment. For we all know innately how powerful and right our intuitive sense is. It is what leads us through most of life's decisions, from choice of profession to choice of lifemate to the basic approach we take to everything from the rearing of children to where to go on vacation. Intuitive knowing is *real* knowing, a thoroughly human kind of knowing. But intuitive insight is wisdom without logical sequence. It does not proceed syllogistically from point A to B. It erupts from within us and more often than not reveals the most important pieces of reality.

It is based on this kind of human knowing that we may reasonably posit God. We find the existence of God and heaven compelling because our intuitive selves, if we will trust them, tell us reality makes no sense otherwise, and we intuitively know also that a nonsensical universe is impossible. Küng has summed this up eloquently:

God's existence is not first proved or demonstrated by reason and then believed, thus guaranteeing the rationality of belief in God. There is not first a rational knowledge and then confident acknowledgement of God. The hidden reality of God is not forced on reason . . . . it is an inward rationality [what I have called intuition] which can offer a fundamental certainty. In the accomplishment, by the "practice" of boldly trusting in God's reality, despite all temptations to doubt, man experiences the reasonableness of his trust.[13]

Perhaps Pascal expressed this even more poetically in his classic epithet, "*Le coeur a ses raisons que la raison ne connaît point*," perhaps fairly translated, "The heart has its reasons of which reason has not the slightest understanding."

I will indict us straight up: our arrogance has led us, through a creature of our own making (science), to imagine that reality consists only of facts of which we have empirical data. Or, if we admit the possibility of other realities, we contend that lacking empirical data, they are not worth tending to. What incredible cheek. What ontological poverty. What a bleak landscape.

Is it any wonder that so much contemporary art and music are devoid of spiritual depth and beauty? We have spawned a universe that does not retreat into mysterious subatomic and all-pervasive energy (in spite of the facts), but into binary bits and bytes through which we have constructed our technocracy at whose magnetic shrine we worship.

But stand, if you will, in the presence of this incomprehensible cosmic energy; stand and gaze upon the incalculable reality of cosmic curvilinear time and space, and tell me—tell me—that you do not faintly make out the face of God, hear the flap of angel wings, or glimpse the gates of heaven. A mode of time that transcends this time, a dimension of space that surpasses anything we know or say of space, are no flights of fancy. Rather, in light of objective inquiry, our intuitive selves compel us to assent to these realities. If we can persuade our usually selective perception to let into our consciousnesses the full reality uncovered by the electron microscope and the cerebral cortices of Albert Einstein and Niels Bohr and Werner Heisenberg and others, I frankly can't imagine that any intelligent being will be unable to hear what Peter Berger has called "a rumor of angels."[14]

# CHAPTER 6

## Affirming the Promise

Heaven and AIDS: what can we say? I would begin by saying to all those of us who are dying (and that includes everyone whose eyes are passing over these words) that it is perfectly reasonable for us to assume that our lives are not contained by our bodies or circumscribed by our births and eventual deaths. We have good reason to expect death to be not an end, but a transition to some different mode of being.

For those of us whose deaths do not appear imminent, the need for this assertion will probably have very little immediacy. At the beginning of my own illness, when I intermittently expected to die, my interest in an afterlife flipped on and off like a toggle switch at precisely those transition points between my thinking I was dying and thinking I was not. I had never realized how potent a force in our psyche rejection of self-annihilation is. I can understand now that the most incomprehensible notion to the human mind is the thought of the end to its own existence. Everything inside of us wells up at the prospect of self-annihilation and shouts, "No, this cannot be. I cannot *not be*." I used to think (as many "death experts" do these days) that this response constituted a bad thing, a lack of acceptance of death. But labeling this response pejoratively would be warranted only if death *were* final for each of our existences. But I contend, and hope I have demonstrated, that trusting our intuition, it is inwardly rational to believe that death is *not* final and that our gut rejection of self-annihilation is simply an accurate reading of reality. I hope that this is of some consolation to my brothers and sisters with AIDS, for whom death is indeed imminent.

It is not that there will be no loss. With every debilitating illness comes loss; anyone with AIDS already has to have experienced this. But there will be more at death; in a sense, dying will involve something of a total loss. All the stuff in your earthly life; all the substance of it including your body will be left behind. And while I cannot speak for you, for all of life's trials I shall miss this earthly life. It has been rich and fascinating. God has done a most excellent job of keeping my life lively. And despite the trouble it has occasionally caused me, I shall also miss what Francis of Assisi called Brother Ass, my body. We have been quite intimate with each other these thirty-nine years. I shall miss its warmth and familiarity.

Death will be no easy parting. So much to say goodbye to. So many friends. So many objects. So much unfinished business. So many unfinished dreams. We shall have grieving to do.

But then, in some way that remains mysterious to us, you and I shall *be* again, or *continue* to be, or be *transformed* into new being, or be *united* with the source of Being: the transmutation defies description. But I am persuaded by all my intuitive power of knowing, affirmed by the wonders revealed by modern scientific inquiry, that at death, life is finished, *but not over*.

This, in itself, is not very satisfying; I assure you that simple ongoing *existence* is not enough for me. As a wise old Benedictine monk once said to me, "If life after death is no more than continued consciousness, who wants it? Who on earth," he continued, "would look forward in joyful expectation to no more than some sort of cosmic merge with the Great Sentience in the Sky to be ever after engaged in being conscious of one's own consciousness? What a bore!" Or as a priest of my acquaintance opened a sermon on heaven by saying, "How many people do you know who say they yearn for everlasting life, but who don't know what to do with themselves on a rainy Sunday afternoon?" As the Benedictine monk concluded, with a confident smile on his face, before walking off with his hands clasped behind his back, "If heaven's not *fuuun*, I'm not goin'!"

So what can we say *qualitatively* about the dimension of existence into which we transcend at death? There are so many people today who claim to have had near-death or out-of-body experiences. The similarity of their experiences is striking. There is always the bright, inviting light; the sense of utter peacefulness and joy; the warmth; and, at the moment of turning back—of being drawn back to this dimension of time and space—the disappointment, the yearning to have continued the transition into everlasting life that was underway.

It is also curious that many of these images and feelings have been expressed in ancient spiritual writings.

The Judeo-Christian Scriptures are full of them. Light is the most prevalent image: "The Lord of Lords, who alone has immortality and dwells in unapproachable light" (1 Tim. 6:16); "The people in darkness have seen a great light" (Matt. 14:16); "God is light and in him is no darkness at all" (1 John 1:5). God has long (long before Christianity) been associated with light or defined as light or, more primitively, as the sun.

Peace and tranquility also commonly are seen as characteristic of the afterlife. "Happy are they who die in the Lord . . . now they can rest forever from their work, since their good deeds go with them" (Rev. 14:13). And joy is always seen as a heavenly state of being: "We rejoice in the hope of sharing the glory of God" (Rom. 5); "Let us not lose sight of Jesus, who leads us in our faith and brings it to perfection; for the sake of the joy which was still in the future, He endured the cross . . . and from now on has taken His place at the right of God's throne" (Heb. 12:2). One could go on.

Are these ancient biblical attributes of the life that transcends death merely pious wishes, projections of the best of all possible human worlds? If so, there is a startling universality about them throughout the breadth and duration of human consciousness. In every world religion that has glimpsed some dimension of being beyond earthly time and space, at least some of these qualities are posited. If they are imaginary, they have all had a remarkable staying power in our imaginations over the millennia.

Finally, I am drawn again to the notions that Jesus

came preaching. You see, there was always this *kingdom* about which He would not stop talking. And it always was both here and not here. "The kingdom of heaven is at hand," He would say, only to say elsewhere, "You are not *far* from the kingdom of God." At the Last Supper, He tells the disciples that the wine He is drinking with them is the last He shall drink with them "until I drink it new in the kingdom of God." In the annunciation story, this kingdom is also closely identified with heaven, since in her vision, Mary hears, "[Your son] will reign over the house of Jacob forever; and of His kingdom, there will be no end" (Luke 1:33). In John's vision, he hears loud voices proclaim, "The kingdom of the world has become the kingdom of our Lord . . . and He shall reign for ever and ever." In the Johannine farewell discourses, Jesus, preparing for His death, tells His disciples, "You are sad now, but I shall see you again, and your hearts will be full of joy, and that joy no one shall take from you" (John 13:22). And finally, in the great priestly prayer, the unitive nature of the kingdom is proclaimed, "May they all be one. Father, may they be one in us, as you are in me and I am in you" (John 17:21).

This is, of course, only a smattering of the heavenly images the Christian Scriptures offer. But they seem to me to touch all the bases. And they are ones with which most readers will be familiar.

What are we to do with all these notions? Even as I chose the preceding passages, I imagined my more rational reader grimacing and saying, "Oh, in the end, he's going to resort to the same old saws." And I simultaneously heard the fundamentalist, finger wagging, condemn me for only offering a *hint* of the inerrant truth of Scripture about all of these things, right down to angels with six wings leaving a few telltale feathers on the floor before me.

In the end, I must make my stand firmly between these two insistent extremes. I will not give up even one Christian metaphor that points toward the mysterious, unnameable, loving reality that we sum up and call God. I will not relinquish them because to do so would isolate me from the deepest levels of truth, a dimension of reality for whose existence there is, I believe, good evidence. We are now more intimately in touch with the wonder of creation than any previous scientific paradigm has made manifest to us. This, coupled with our own trustworthy intuition, makes quite reasonable the expectation of heaven.

I am not much interested in dwelling in a technological vacuum, even if it would be convenient. I reject this ghetto. Creation is too full, reality too pregnant, to be confined by a bits-and-bytes technocracy. I will not opt for the impoverishment of twentieth-century scientism. And so I will not treat these metaphors as so many instances of human imaginary genius. I claim that they point to realities.

On the other hand, I will not confuse metaphor with reality. What is true need not be factual. I do not believe anyone named Eve ever had a set-to with a snake. I do not believe Jesus is a lamb seated on a throne with a zillion eyes and a sword sticking out of His mouth. And I do not believe heaven looks like the Emerald City of Oz.

And so I shall have to rest content in this earthly mode of my existence with only a *rumor* of angels. It would be tempting, for psychological relief, to slide toward scientism or biblical literalism. It would be comforting. But the price would be too high: it would require my sanity either way. For to deny the fullness of reality in order to fit comfortably into a technological universe would constitute a kind of practiced schizophrenia; and, on the other side, to live in a fairy-tale world of children's Bible stories would be even more patently psychotic.

I would like to end with a clear statement of my faith concerning heaven. For in the face of thousands of my sisters and brothers dying of this voracious disease called AIDS, my final desire is to comfort, but with *real* comfort. And so I shall say this:

I believe that my life here is only a kind of holograph, a projection of the fullness of life that I simply cannot trace back in any definitive way to its source.

I believe that the fullness of life of which I speak emanates from a dimension of reality not confined by time and space as we know them; if time and space have any meaning at all in that realm, they are boundless, both implosively so that each moment contains the totality of all moments and explosively so that a trillion infinities could not contain them.

I believe that I dwell in that realm *now*; that the kingdom is immanent, in our midst, among us. It is the source of all that is; it keeps all in existence; it resounds through all matter, giving it being. But I catch only glimpses of this dimension. The trees of our earthly life blind us to the cosmic forest. The stuff of *daily* life makes opaque to us the reality of *eternal* life.

I believe this kingdom shall have no end, no end of peace or joy or rest or comfort or light, although, while all these words intimate the wonderful giftedness of this dimension of being called heaven, we cannot know what any of such metaphors mean in that context. They are all only signposts, not the place itself.

I believe it is into the fullness of this heavenly dimension of being that I shall be transmuted when I die. And I look forward to it, not that this life will have been regrettable, for all its pain and suffering, which can be great. No, I shall look forward to heaven because it seems to me where life naturally leads. This mode of existence *yearns* for a conclusion.

All of which leads to the capstone of my beliefs, namely, that this heaven for which I yearn will mean dwelling fully in the presence of God, God who is infinitely caring, lovingly embracing all that She creates, benevolent and boundless in Her love. And I believe more that He is forthcoming, active, inviting, enticing. It is to this divine invitation that I most want to respond. It is fully with God that I yearn to dwell.

And in light of these beliefs, I can pray for myself, with my chronic affliction; I can pray with all my fellow creatures, who must contend with the various distresses of their lives; but especially at this time would

I pray with my brothers and sisters with AIDS. And my prayer is this:

Almighty God, in your own good time, bring us home to the fullness of joy and peace and oneness that you have promised us. Bring us home, O Loving One, to that peace which is beyond our understanding. Lead us to that place where you shall wipe away every tear, where death shall be no more, and where there shall be neither mourning nor crying nor pain any more, but where we shall dwell with you in unfathomable light.

Without the hope of this promise, life's end would be the bleakest of realities. I cannot prove the truth of eternal life to you. But if you are in need of its comfort at this moment, I tell you that I trust this promise with my whole heart and soul, mind and body. And I share with you my conviction that unending joy awaits you . . . and me. Soon enough.

See you when I get home, my friend.

Godspeed.

# Notes

Chapter 1: From the Bottom of the Heap

1. John E. Fortunato, *Embracing the Exile: Healing Journeys of Gay Christians* (New York: The Seabury Press, 1982).
2. Robin Scroggs, *The New Testament and Homosexuality: Contextual Background for Contemporary Debate* (Philadelphia: Fortress Press, 1983).
3. John Boswell, *Christianity, Social Tolerance, and Homosexuality* (Chicago: University of Chicago, 1980).
4. John MacQuarrie, *The Principles of Christian Theology, 2d ed.* (New York: Scribner & Sons, 1977), 12.
5. *New York Times*, 9 September, 1986, Science Times Section, 19–20.
6. Tom Shealey, "The United States vs. the World: How We Score in Health," *Prevention*, May 1986, 68–72.
7. More precisely, 55 percent are Protestant, 38 percent Catholic, and 3 percent Eastern Orthodox, according to the *World Book Encyclopaedia* (Chicago, 1986), 20:58.
8. Howard Brown, *Familiar Faces, Hidden Lives: The Story of Homosexual Men in America Today* (New York: Harcourt Brace Jovanovich, 1976) contains many stories about how this "skill" is learned.
9. I recommend Ram Dass's *Journey of Awakening: A Meditator's Guidebook* (New York: Bantam Books, 1978) as a good "translation" of Eastern meditative practice for Western use.
10. Gerald G. May's book *Simply Sane: Stop Fixing Yourself and Start Really Living* (New York: Paulist Press, 1977) is the best antidote I know to spiritual "works-ism."
11. Barry Stevens, *Don't Push the River (It Flows by Itself)* (Lafayette, CA: Real People Press, 1970).
12. Christopher Lasch, *The Culture of Narcissism: American Life in an Age of Diminishing Expectations* (New York: Norton, 1978) paints a clear picture of this aspect of contemporary society.

13. *Psychology Today*, May 1983, 13, graph.
14. Lillene Fifield, "Alcoholism and the Gay Community," a synopsis of a report published by the Gay Community Services Center, Los Angeles, California, entitled, "On My Way to Nowhere: Alienated, Isolated, Drunk; An Analysis of Gay Alcohol Abuse and an Evaluation of Alcoholism Rehabilitation Services in the Los Angeles Gay Community" (1975) (synopsis, unpublished, available from author, 856 N.E. Oakland, Roseburg, OR 97470).

Chapter 2: Disembodiment: The Orthodox Heresy

1. This word in common parlance has come to have a slightly erotic flavor. I do not mean it in that way at all. *Sensuous* here means only that which is taken in by the senses—that is, that which is seen, smelled, tasted, heard, or touched. But the word does connote worldliness, because it is through the senses that we let in the world.
2. D. M. Baillie, *God Was in Christ: An Essay on Incarnation and Atonement* (New York: Charles Scribner's Sons, 1948), 11.
3. Bede Griffiths, *The Marriage of East and West* (Springfield, IL: Templegate Press, 1982), 109.
4. Kenneth E. Kirk, *The Vision of God: The Christian Doctrine of the Summum Bonum* (London: Longmans, Green and Co., 1931), 312ff.
5. Kenneth E. Kirk, *Vision of God*, 177–178.
6. Chapman Cohen, *Religion and Sex: Studies in the Pathology of Religious Development* (New York: AMS Press, 1975), 122.
7. *The Hymnal of the Protestant Episcopal Church in the United States of America* (New York: Church Pension Fund, 1940), nos. 301, 197, and 136.
8. William E. Phipps, *Recovering Biblical Sensuousness* (Philadelphia: Westminster Press, 1975) provides an excellent account of this whole topic.
9. *TANAKH: A New Translation of the Holy Scriptures According to the Traditional Hebrew Text* (Philadelphia: Jewish Publication Society, 1985), 1405–17.
10. Bernard de Clairvaux, *On the Song of Songs, 1* and *On the Song of Songs, 2* in *The Works of Bernard of Clairvaux* (Spencer, MA: Cistercian Publications, 1970).

11. Reginald Fuller, from a lecture delivered at the Virginia Theological Seminary in 1974.

12. James E. Nelson, *Embodiment: An Approach to Sexuality and Christian Theology* (Minneolis: Augsburg, 1978).

Chapter 3: The Dilemma

1. The recent increase in violence against gay people and its relationship to AIDS was well documented in an ABC "20/20" segment aired nationally on April 10, 1986.

2. Edward Shils, *Tradition* (Chicago: University of Chicago Press, 1981), 221–22.

3. Karl Rahner, *Foundations of Christian Faith: An Introduction to the Idea of Christianity* (New York: Seabury Press, 1978), 271.

4. Lloyd "Ben" Kemena, "AIDS Patient Stirs Emotions of Love, Hate," *Chicago Tribune*, 27 April 1986, sec. 3, p. 1., col. 1.

Chapter 4: Bearing the Pain

1. This valuable piece of wisdom was given me by Dr. Gerald G. May of the Shalem Institute for Spiritual Formation.

2. Isshu Miura and Ruth Fuller Sasaki, *Zen Dust: The History of the Koan and Koan Study in Rinzai (Lin-Chi) Zen* (New York: Brace & World, 1966), 7. First koan from 121.

3. The last three koans taken from Diasetz Teitaro Suzuki, *An Introduction to Zen Buddhism* (New York: Grove Press, 1964), 59.

4. John Hick, *Evil and the God of Love* (New York: Harper & Row, 1966) is the most thorough treatment of this topic I have read.

5. Susan Simmons-Alling, "AIDS: Psychosocial Needs of the Health Care Worker," *Topics in Clinical Nursing* (July 1984): 31.

6. *Diagnostic and Statistical Manual of Mental Disorders,* 3d ed. (Washington, DC: American Psychiatric Association, 1980), 380.

7. Marilyn Chase, "The AIDS Business: Drug Firms Anticipate Big Market in Products for Immune Disorder," *Wall Street Journal*, 26 June, 1986, 1.

8. Harold S. Kushner, *When Bad Things Happen to Good People* (New York: Schocken Books, 1981).

9. C. S. Lewis, *The Problem of Pain* (New York: Macmillan, 1962), 110.

10. Recollected from a sermon preached by the Rev. Alison M. Cheek at St. Stephen and the Incarnation Church, Washington, D.C.
11. Elisabeth Kübler-Ross, *On Death and Dying* (New York: Macmillan, 1969).
12. Examples include Gen. 18:22–33; Gen. 32:24–32; Exod. 3:13ff., 4:1ff., 4:10ff.; Exod. 32:11ff.
13. John 13:5–9
14. Pierre Wolff, *May I Hate God?* (New York: Paulist Press, 1966), 57.
15. Lewis, *Problem of Pain*, 10.
16. O'Kelley Whitaker, *Sister Death* (New York: Morehouse-Barlow, 1974).
17. Sister Patrice Murphy's article "Pastoral Care and Persons with AIDS: A Means to Alleviate Physical, Emotional, Social and Spiritual Suffering," published in the *American Journal of Hospice Care* (March-April 1986), 38, is the most open, clear, grounded invitation to love PWAs in practical ways I have read.

Chapter 5: A Case for Heaven

1. C. S. Lewis, *The Problem of Pain* (New York: Macmillan, 1962), 144.
2. *A Mencken Chrestomathy*, ed. and annot., H.L. Mencken (NY: Vintage Books, 1982), 91.
3. Gary Zukav, *The Dancing Wu Li Masters: An Overview of the New Physics* (New York: William Morrow, 1979), 23.
4. W. Heisenberg, *Across the Frontiers* (New York: Harper & Row, 1974).
5. Hans Küng, *Does God Exist? An Answer for Today* (Garden City, NY: Doubleday, 1978), 460ff.
6. W. Stegmüller, from *Metaphysik, Skepsis, Wissenschaft*, quoted in Küng, *Does God Exist?*, 461.
7. Küng, *Does God Exist?*, 462.
8. John Bertram Phillips, *Your God Is Too Small* (New York: Macmillan, 1953).
9. John Gribbin, *In Search of Schrödinger's Cat: Quantum Physics and Reality* (Toronto: Bantam, 1984), 235–236.
10. Marilyn Ferguson, *The Aquarian Conspiracy: Personal and Social Transformation in the 1980s* (Los Angeles: J.P. Tarcher, 1980).
11. Küng, *Does God Exist?*, 571.

12. Carl Gustav Jung, *Psychological Types* (Princeton, NJ: Princeton University Press, 1971).
13. Küng, *Does God Exist?*, 574.
14. Peter L. Berger, *A Rumor of Angels: Modern Sociology and the Rediscovery of the Supernatural* (Garden City, NY: Doubleday, 1969).